THE REAL CURE

Healing Essentials, LLC

ISBN 979-8-9989922-0-9

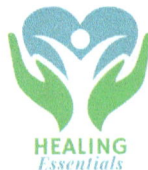

THE REAL CURE

Wisdom from a Traditional Naturopath

By Cynthia L Maguire, ND, CTN, CBS

Testimonials

"A couple of years ago, I had a gallbladder attack that sent me to the ER followed by a consultation with a surgeon. I decided to investigate ways that might help me keep my gallbladder as my mother suffered with diarrhea after her gallbladder was taken out. My cousin had been seeing Dr. Cynthia Maguire and had very positive experiences with her, so I decided to reach out. It was the best decision ever to connect with Dr. Cynthia! Not only has she helped me with my gallbladder, but also so many other things! Blood work taken by my regular doctor turned a corner within six months. Concerning issues with my kidneys were completely dissolved! I believe she will keep me on the right track to a healthier life."

~ Brenda R.

"Cynthia Maguire has been working with my husband and myself for several years and has helped us solve several different issues in our lives. She is very thorough and understands the body so very well and knows what causes certain issues and helps us to resolve them. I can't thank her enough for all she has done for us with her wonderful expertise in so many ways. I highly recommend Cynthia as a Naturopath."

~ Patti M.

"Early in 2017, I was informed I had prostate cancer. My PSA numbers were high enough to create concern. After discussion with a surgeon and a radiologist to explore what seemed to be imminent, my wife and I sought for another means, a natural way to fight cancer. Cynthia has been a blessing from the start of our journey together. Since meeting with Cynthia, I elected to be on active surveillance and forego surgery or radiation treatment. With Cynthia's expertise as a Naturopath, her supplement suggestions along with a modified diet and continued exercise, I was able to maintain daily vitality and keep my cancer in check for over five years before finally electing to surgically remove the cancer. Cynthia and her God given expertise definitely helped my wife and I navigate through these trials."

~ Tim M.

"I have had the privilege of visiting as a client and learning from Cynthia Maguire, a highly skilled and knowledgeable naturopath for over 20 years. Her expertise in utilizing herbs and essential oils is truly remarkable, and her ability to share this knowledge through her client care and training sessions is inspiring. Cynthia's passion for holistic wellness shines through in everything she does, making her an invaluable resource for anyone seeking to learn about natural healing methods. She brings professionalism, clarity, and a deep understanding to her work, leaving a lasting impact on everyone she works with."

~ Katrina R.

DEDICATION

This book is dedicated to my beloved husband, James J. Maguire, and our four children; Michelle Tyre, Misty Auckerman, Nathaniel Castilla and Kimberly Clark. My precious family has encouraged me for years to write this book about my cleansing process, along with the wisdom I have gleaned over the last 30 years as a Traditional Naturopath. I also dedicate this book to the numerous clients and colleagues who have been waiting for this work to be accomplished. Last, but certainly not least, I dedicate this book to my God, who has dramatically changed my life and partnered with me all along the way, teaching me, encouraging me and guiding me to bring this information to the public. I love you all. You are so very dear to my heart!

Sincerely,

Cynthia L Maguire, ND, CTN, CBS

Healing Essentials, LLC

DISCLAIMER

The information contained in this book is for educational purposes only. It is not provided to diagnose, prescribe, or treat. The information in this book should not be used as a substitute for medical counseling with a health professional. Neither the author nor publisher accept responsibility for such use.

***

I will also be mentioning two brand names of products you may choose to use. These are the two main companies I use in helping my clients due to the high quality and potency of their products. Following are links to these companies that will enable you to get a free wholesale account, of which I will receive a small dividend when products are purchased. These are just suggestions. Please feel free to use whatever products you feel are appropriate.

- doTERRA: referral.doterra.me/395170

- Nature's Sunshine Products (NSP): naturessunshine.com/ referrer=197907&offer=NSP&cid=other

***

An excellent way to rid the body of environmental and heavy metal toxins, as well as fungi and parasites, is to invest in an ion cleanse detoxification system. My husband, James J Maguire, DAC, CBS, promotes an excellent one that is superior, for a number of reasons, to most others on the market. The IonCleanse by AMD is a safer medical grade piece of equipment that does not generate any unwanted negative electromagnetic energy, as do other units. The toxins in the body have either a positive or negative electrical charge. Cheap units only generate negative ions to cleanse the body of positively charged toxins, providing half the needed cleanse. The Ion Cleanse by AMD employs a more advanced and sophisticated technology, capable of generating both positive and negative ions for the most thorough and complete cleanse possible.

Check out his website at jamesjmaguire.com. Click on the link for "Products" and look for the IonCleanse. It would be a very wise investment for you and your family. On his web site, you can also find electromagnetic frequency (EMF) protection devices, as well as some other great products for natural health care.

CONTENTS

PART 3: THE PROCESS

PROLOGUE

I was born and raised in the lush farmland of the Midwest in Springfield, Ohio. My mother's family had their roots in the mountains of West Virginia, hill folk from the Appalachian Mountains. If you are ever curious about what kind of people they were, the book *Hillbilly Elegy* by J.D. Vance hits the nail right on the head. They were a mixed group of people descended from Scots-Irish and Buffalo Ridge Cherokees from Virginia. My mom had a ninth-grade education and married at the age of 17, which was common among hill folk. But what she lacked in schooling, she made up for in good-old survival skills. I grew up eating garden fresh veggies, eggs straight from the chickens, meat from hens that had grown too old to lay eggs, rabbits (that we dared not turn into pets), and beef and pork from the farm animals my dad raised and slaughtered. He was also a trapper, so we ate a lot of wild game as well: snapping turtles, squirrels, muskrats, gophers, and other critters I wouldn't dream of eating now.

I loved helping my family plant the garden, then waiting and watching for the baby plants to pop their heads up out of the soil. I learned to identify their leaves pretty quickly. I also learned to identify a lot of other plants on the farm, like nettles, poison ivy, and poison oak. If you've ever wandered into a patch of these, I'm sure, like me, you will never want to forget what they look like!

My mom and grandmother taught me to can and freeze veggies and berries (we made amazing jams and jellies), so we always had enough food stored for the winter. While we canned, Grandma told me tales of her father and how he would hunt and trap in the woods and bring home medicinal plants. He also had a pet raccoon, who followed him around everywhere.

Though we always found a way to make ends meet, trips to the store for candy and sweets were a luxury we definitely couldn't afford. This was a good thing in the long run because we had strong, healthy teeth. We took care of most of our health concerns with love, time, patience, and home-made chicken noodle soup. A doctor was called only for the most serious of injuries: a broken bone or a wound needing stitches. Vaccinations at that time were minimal. Cod liver oil, followed by a healthy dose of peanut butter, was a daily norm, especially in the winter. In the springtime, the doctor would have us take these little red pills for parasites and mom would spend the day changing all of the bed sheets, sweeping and mopping the floors, and cleaning the bathrooms and mattresses. I now understand the wisdom of this routine, which is something doctors and mothers of today have nearly forgotten.

When I was 16, I secured a job at Wright-Patterson AFB Headquarters as a secretary. By the age of 35, I was working full-time, raising four children, and going to college during my lunch break. I was studying business courses, hoping to move up the ladder at work. Then, one fateful day, my whole life took a new and unexpected direction.

I had just picked up my two youngest children from school and was stopped, waiting to make a left turn. Suddenly, a large white van going about 50 mph slammed into the right rear of my station wagon, catapulting us into the other lane of traffic, where we were hit head on by a large Cadillac that was also going about 50 mph.

Thank God, everyone survived; only a few minor surgeries were needed, but I suffered a severe case of whiplash. The tormenting pain in my neck and shoulders propelled me into a year-long search for relief. The doctors tried everything they knew how to do in order to alleviate the pain, using several different prescriptions and types of therapy, including: massage, traction, chiropractic treatments, trigger point therapy, and nearly 50 cortisone shots into the small knots that persisted in the muscles of my shoulders. Each new treatment brought only brief moments of relief before the pain returned. I was in constant agony.

After a year of frustration, anger, and exhaustion, a friend of mine recommended seeing a more "natural" doctor. Why not? I thought. Nothing else had worked, so I decided to give it a try. After asking me a few questions, he did something he called muscle testing and determined that I should try potassium and St. John's Wort. He explained that my muscles needed a lot more potassium to help them relax. He also explained that even though St. John's Wort was useful for supporting a healthy mental attitude, it was also useful to help soothe frayed nerve endings. I started his protocol, and, after only a few weeks, I woke up one morning to discover that my neck and shoulders had completely relaxed! I was thrilled! I couldn't believe it had worked and thought it was probably just a fluke and wouldn't last. The good news was, it did!

A few weeks later, I was back in the emergency room with excruciating pain in my lower right groin. I thought I might be having an appendicitis attack, but when I hopped up on the table, the pain miraculously disappeared. I felt really foolish and embarrassed. I told the doctor I was fine and that for some reason the pain was gone. They checked my appendix anyway, and it was fine. Then they checked my kidneys for stones. When the emergency room physician gave me the results of my X-rays, he told me that I had so many kidney stones that they couldn't even count them. I evidently had a stone stuck in my right ureter, and when I hopped up onto the table, the slight jarring dislodged the stone and it passed into my bladder, relieving me of pain. I immediately thought about my grandfather. He had a jar of kidney stones that doctors had removed. Many were the size of regular marbles, while some were the size of shooter marbles. He eventually died from kidney failure after being on dialysis for several months. It was extremely scary to think I might be going down the same path.

The hospital doctor talked about the procedure they would use to shatter the kidney stones. Since I would be passing the shards for a while and it would be extremely painful, they would have to keep me at the hospital on pain meds until I had passed all of them. Since I was no longer in pain, I told the hospital to release me, and I would think about it and let them know. What they wanted to do would entail several days of being off work, with no one at home to help with my four small children.

I went back to see the Naturopathic Doctor and asked him if there was anything he could do for kidney stones. He did some more muscle testing and told me he would recommend hydrangea and lecithin, then explained the dosage I needed. He sent me home to strain my urine and said to call him if I saw anything. Within about a week and a half, I started seeing squishy yellow globules coming out with my urine. I called him and told him what I was seeing. He said that those were what kidney stones looked like after the hydrangea and lecithin had softened them up. In the end, I passed 42 globules. Needless to say, my kidney doctor was astonished when he ran the test again and found everything clear.

I was so impressed by my recent experiences that I went back to the Naturopathic Doctor. I told him I didn't understand what he did, but I was fascinated and wanted to learn what he knew. It had become my dream to help others the way he had helped me. I asked if he would teach me, and he agreed.

I switched my major in college to the sciences and did an understudy with him for nearly four years. One of the things he taught me was how to do an advanced form of muscle testing called Contact Reflex Analysis (CRA). I finished my Bachelor of Science degree at the local college and started studying at Clayton College, completing a Master's Degree in Herbology and a Doctorate in Naturopathy. It took 15 years of studying part-time to complete all of this while raising my four children, mostly alone. It was hard, but it was definitely the most well-spent 15 years of my life. I was the first one in my family to ever attend college and the first to get a doctorate, something of which my mother was extremely proud.

During my 30 years in practice, I have had the opportunity to muscle test hundreds of clients. While I was doing all that testing, there were some important things that became very apparent. I was able to figure out the root cause of many health issues, as well as a series of cleanses that could get at those root causes. I also learned that there was a definite protocol to follow while doing the cleanses so that I didn't make my clients feel even worse during the healing process.

During the first few years of my practice, instead of cleansing, I would give my clients products that would support their various health issues. For example, I would give my clients *Uva-Ursi*, or *Buchu* to support their kidneys. This would help as long as the client was on the product. But, as soon as I stopped the product, their urinary problems would return. I quickly realized that if I did not eliminate the root cause of their kidney issues, such as kidney stones, yeast or urinary parasites, I was fighting a losing battle. Once I had them do the cleanses for the various root problems of the urinary system, I could then wean them off of the supporting products, and their kidney issues would not return.

As I helped my clients through their cleansing and rebuilding process, their regular doctors began to reduce and even eliminate many prescription drugs. At the same time, my clients were gaining strength, energy, and vitality.

In the 17th Century, many people who were skilled in the use of herbs for healing were branded as witches. Fortunately, since those dark ages, modern science has helped us to understand the practice of both herbology and muscle testing. Pharmacopeia has given us many modern medicines based on the healing properties found in herbs. Muscle testing, also branded as voodoo, has been vindicated by quantum physics, which helps us understand that anything, when introduced into an energy field, can increase or decrease the strength of that energy field. This can be determined on a human by doing a simple muscle test. Therefore, being backed by modern science, I proudly and officially stake my claim as an unapologetic "witch doctor."

PART 1
THE BASICS

1

CONFRONTING THE MESS

Daren unlocked the door to the old woman's house. She was a recluse and had passed away quite a while ago. Daren had been handed the duty of clearing up her estate. It was obvious when he pulled up that the property was in bad need of attention. The lawn was overgrown and the walkway leading up to the door was barely visible through the choking weeds.

He cautiously cracked open the door. The smell that hit his nose was so strong it made him take a few steps back. His hand automatically searched for the mask and bottle of lavender he had tucked in his pocket. He put a generous amount on the mask and quickly donned it, grateful for his loving wife, who had insisted that he bring it along. This was going to be quite an experience.

Daren pushed the door open and peered inside. A couple of mice, startled by his presence, quickly scampered across the sofa and disappeared under a dusty pillow. Old books and magazines were piled everywhere. Moldy, rotting food lay on the coffee table, along with a half-full soda that was feeding a swarm of flies. Dust covered everything.

He made his way to the kitchen, noticing a few webs that hosted spiders who were enjoying a snack. Empty containers of take-out food lay strewn around. Dishes were piled high on the counters and stacked deep in a sink full of stagnant water.

Several roaches noticed his unwelcome presence and quickly dashed off the counter to find a good hiding spot. The table was barely visible under the mounds of mail, along with still more moldy containers of unrecognizable take-out food. The horrible smell was threatening to seep past all that lavender on his mask, so he quickly dabbed a few more drops on it. He inched his way over to the refrigerator and opened it, then winced and quickly shut it as the pungent fumes stung his eyes.

He decided to move past that mess and made his way to the bedroom. Clothes were strewn across every available surface, including the floor. Books and magazines were piled high in every nook and cranny. The stench was even more overwhelming in the bedroom. It smelled like something was rotting somewhere. Then he spied the bathroom door. He wondered if he even dared to look in there. Carefully making his way across the littered floor, he reached the door to the bathroom and cracked it open. The sight and smell that assaulted his senses was unbelievable. The toilet had overflowed, with feces spilling on the floor, where a swarm of flies and maggots were feasting. Fearing he would vomit, Daren fled for the front door.

Once again in the fresh air, he ripped off his mask and grabbed his stomach. His mind raced. *Unbelievable! How could anyone live like that? How in the world will I get this mess cleaned up and the house ready for sale? Where do I even begin?*

***

Now, can you now imagine what it would be like if we took care of our homes the way we take care of our health? People think about cleaning their homes, their offices, their desks, their cars, their yards, their closets, and even their septic tanks — but how many times do you hear people talking about cleaning out their bodies? What do you think happens when you don't have regular bowel movements or your kidneys, liver, gallbladder, and arteries get clogged up with undissolved debris? Just like the trash in our homes attracts maggots and other unwanted creepy-crawly things, the trash and debris in our bodies attract parasites, fungi, and an accumulation of harmful chemicals that wreak havoc on our health. The body's various organ systems begin to back up and shut down. Little by little, we lose vitality and quickly age.

The solution to the problem is to focus on preventive maintenance. Our current healthcare system operates as a business. Healthcare providers focus on suppression of symptoms, not preventive maintenance. Businesses, doctors, hospitals, pharmaceutical companies, and insurance firms need to make money, but they don't make money when patients are healthy. Prevention is not in their best interest, so what they do is merely suppress symptoms. For instance, most arthritis medications are really just painkillers. They may help take away the pain, but they certainly don't take away the arthritis. This is a very short-sighted system for a suffering patient. The BIG FOUR concerns of heart disease, cancer, stroke, and diabetes account for about 83% of all deaths, but are mostly lifestyle diseases born of poor choices.

To make matters worse, prescription drugs are causing serious side-effects. The Centers for Disease Control (CDC) estimates that more than 20 million unnecessary prescriptions for antibiotics are handed out each year. Currently, more than 95% of staph bacteria are resistant to penicillin. MRSA is now causing more deaths in the U.S. than AIDS (Journal of American Medical Association). There are 2.2 million cases of adverse reactions related to prescription drugs each year. Close to two million hospitalized patients fall victim to hospital-acquired infections (HAIs) annually, resulting in nearly 100,000 hospital deaths each year. This exceeds the number of deaths from AIDS, breast cancer, and automobile accidents combined.

We need to get back to the basics. We need a healthy diet with proper nutrition, appropriate exercise, correct posture, regular deep breathing, adequate water intake, the cleansing of vermin and toxins from our bodies, and the elimination of mental toxins from our minds.

Aging begins at the cellular level. Toxins in the body create stress, which leads to cellular inflammation. When we first receive an injury or an infection, inflammation is a critically important and necessary part of the healing process. The instant we experience an injury or the invasion of a harmful microbe, inflammatory chemicals marshal a defensive attack, laying waste to harmful invaders and to any infected tissue. Once the attack is over, inflammation subsides and the cleansing and healing process begins.

However, if the body's inflammatory response becomes chronic, it sets up an environment for our most deadly and chronic diseases, such as diabetes, cardiovascular disease, arthritis, auto-immune disorders, various neurological diseases, and cancer.

When a cell becomes inflamed, the major cellular transport system shuts down. No nutrients can get in and no waste can get out. The cell then becomes too weak to sufficiently hold its boundaries and eventually spills out its contents and dies. However, sometimes if the DNA has mutated, the cell forgets how to die and instead becomes cancerous.

When our bodies have become dis-eased, where do we begin? This is the question I get from most of my new clients: I know I need to cleanse my body, but where do I start? In the next chapters, we will discuss health basics. Then I will pull it all together for you so you will know how to safely and properly cleanse: where to start, how to proceed, and some suggestions of natural products to use in the process. I am also going to delve a little into mental health and the science of psychoneuroimmunology. But first, I am going to teach you how to accurately muscle test so you will have a tool to help you figure out exactly what you need to do and how to do it.

2
MUSCLE TESTING

The real cure to our healthcare crisis is for people to have the
knowledge and tools to take better care of themselves.
~ James J. Maguire, DAC, CBS

When I was first introduced to muscle testing, I thought it was really weird. If you have ever experienced it, you probably felt the same way. How could my doctor just hand me something, or say something, and my arm would automatically be strong or go weak regardless of what I was thinking or how hard I tried to resist the downward pressure? It made no sense at all. What I did know, however, is that muscle testing gave him the information he needed to correctly recommend the products and dosages I needed to heal, even when no other treatment or therapy had worked. It not only worked the first time to release my whiplash, but it also worked the second time to help break down and release the kidney stones. It may have seemed weird, but it was also a miracle. It worked, and I wanted to learn how it was done and why it worked.

After my first experience with muscle testing, I attended a couple of weekend seminars where I learned how to do basic muscle testing and an advanced form of muscle testing called Contact Reflex Analysis. I also learned a lot about the history of muscle testing and the different methods used. Since then, I have taught muscle testing in many one-day seminars to both professionals and non-professionals. Yes, a one-day seminar is all it takes to learn the basics, but to become accurate takes a lot of practice.

Muscle testing is a branch of a broader science called kinesiology. Basically, it is the art of applying consistent force to a muscle in the presence of a stimulus, then observing the response of whether the muscle stays strong or goes weak.

During the classes I taught, students would often begin debating over which method was the most proper way to do muscle testing. These debates caused me to look into the history of kinesiology to find out why there were so many differing opinions on the subject. In a nutshell, this is what I learned:

- In the 1940s, Henry and Florence Kendall, MSA SC, pioneered the development of kinesiology. This method was a strictly clinical procedure to determine the strength and weakness of specific muscles in order to treat the injured ones. They were best known for their work with polio patients.

- In the 1950s, Richard Versendaal, DC, founded Contact Reflex Analysis (CRA). He discovered 75 major energy points on the body that can be touched while muscle testing to determine physical imbalances.

- In the 1960s Alan Beardall, DC, founded Clinical Kinesiology (CK). He discovered that certain hand modes (e.g., touching the thumb with one of the other fingers of that same hand) affected muscle testing.

- In 1964, George Goodheart, DC, founded Applied Kinesiology (AK), combining Eastern ideas about energy flow with Western ideas about muscle testing. He also linked muscle weakness to specific glands and organs, as well as substances.

- In 1979, John Diamond, MD, published his book, titled Behavioral Kinesiology, linking muscle strength with emotional and intellectual stimuli.

- In 1984, Solihin Thom, DO, expanded kinesiology into the realm of human consciousness and called it Ontological Kinesiology (OK), which he now calls Inner Dialogue™.

- In 1995, David Hawkins, MD, PhD, published Power Vs. Force, in which he created the Christ Consciousness Scale and used muscle testing to determine both the truthfulness of information and our own consciousness level.

***

As you can see, many models of kinesiology or muscle testing have been developed over the years. Moreover, modern science is just beginning to scratch the surface of the mystery of quantum physics and how the human energy field is affected by different types of energy.

In the entanglement theory, quantum physics gives us the clearest answers as to why muscle testing works.

Some simplified energy facts are:

- Everything in the universe is made up of vibrating energy.

- Energy vibrations can either enhance or decrease each other, or remain neutral.

- Words and thoughts create their own energy vibrations.

- The vibration of a truth causes the energy field to be strengthened and elicits a strong muscle response, while the vibration of a lie weakens the energy field and elicits a weak muscle response.

**

I love knowing that the vibration of truth strengthens us. This verifies to me that we have an innate God-given ability to sense right from wrong, true from false, and good from bad. Essentially, anything that is good, right, or true for us strengthens our core energy, while anything bad, wrong, or false for us weakens our core energy. If we become keenly in tune with our energy field, spirit, feelings, and intuition, we can know the correct path to take in our lives, the correct substances to consume, and whether other people are telling us the truth or trying to pull the wool over our eyes.

**

I have used and taught muscle testing for nearly 30 years now, and have learned that there are several rules that should be followed for the most reliable muscle testing:

1. There should be two people (the tester and the testee) for the most accurate muscle testing. You can muscle test yourself, but you could be prejudiced in your thoughts, thereby skewing the results. So having a second person available will make the testing more accurate, assuming they are not prejudiced toward a certain outcome as well.

2. The consciousness level of the person being tested must be at least 200 (see the Christ Consciousness Scale in David Hawkins book, *Power Vs. Force*). Anyone that has a consciousness level below 200 is literally incapable of knowing truth from falsehood or right from wrong. This would involve cases where people are extremely mentally challenged or when people, such as sociopaths and other criminals, have become incapable of knowing right from wrong. In this case a surrogate needs to be used.

3. One muscle should be isolated as much as possible while muscle testing. Using the forearm is often the most accurate way to test. To test using only the forearm, have the person stand with their arm hanging down at their side then have them just raise their forearm parallel to the floor, keeping their upper arm next to their side. Then apply pressure at the wrist with your fingers or hand. Using the entire arm out to the side is commonly used, but this method has two flaws. One, it is very tiring for the testee and they are likely to become weaker and more easily give false negatives. Second, it involves several different muscles which can be used to compensate for weakness.

4. There must be consistent force and resistance applied to the muscle. The tester should not push down gently and slowly one time, then push quickly and harshly the second. Pushing gently and slowly will offer the most accurate results. Also, the person being tested must not be in a weakened position by having already been muscle tested too long. A young child, a person who has a shoulder injury, or a person who has a disability in their shoulders must be able to have enough strength to be tested. If not,

10

use a surrogate. When a surrogate is needed, use another person as the testee for the client. You will muscle test the arm of the surrogate as you ask questions or make statements about the client. You must have permission from the person being tested to ask the questions, especially if the person being asked about is not present. If the person being the surrogate is the parent or legal guardian of the one being tested, permission is assumed. Also, if you are the legal medical representative of an unconscious person, permission is also assumed. Surrogate testing for information about an adult who is capable of being tested themselves is an invasion of privacy and against the laws of the universe. In this case, you are unlikely to receive accurate answers.

5. If the person being tested is present, have the surrogate and the client hold hands or touch in some other way, or, if it is a rambunctious toddler being tested, have the parent stay intently focused on the child.

6. If testing someone at a distance through a surrogate, make the strongest energetic connection possible. For example, make a phone call to the person being tested and have them stay on the phone while you are testing or use a picture that both you and the surrogate can focus on. If possible, use a relative or close friend to be the surrogate of the testee.

7. The proper polarity of the tester and the testee must be functioning. To test for proper polarity, point a finger in the area between the eyes in alignment with the eyebrows. You do not need to physically touch this area. Just bring your finger within an inch of the skin. Once the finger is in place, prompt the person to hold out their arm, prompt

them to resist your pressure, then press down on the forearm with a slow steady pressure. The arm should go weak and not be able to resist the pressure. If the arm does not go weak, then their polarity is reversed. This can be corrected by making sure the testee is well-hydrated and by having the testee do brain gym exercises.

Brain Gym Exercises

Crossover exercises (repeatedly raising the right knee while touching it with the left hand, then raising the left knee while touching it with the right hand).

Walking in a figure eight pattern from both directions.

Focused breathing (focusing on running energy up the back with the in-breath and down the front with the out-breath).

---

8. If these exercises do not work, then have some of the herb spirulina on hand and have them take four capsules with a glass of water and wait a few minutes. If all of this fails, you can then proceed to test them, knowing that everything will be the exact opposite of what the truth is. True statements will make them go weak and false statements will make them go strong. Substances they need will make them go weak and substances they don't need will make them go strong. The world is a very confusing place for people whose polarity is reversed. Their intuition is continually backwards. There are several main causes for someone's polarity to be reversed, such as dehydration, contamination with toxic heavy metals, and the constant bombardment of their energy field with electro-magnetic

frequencies from things like cell phones, computers, electrical wiring, etc. Their polarity can be corrected over time with the proper adjustments.

9. Remove all large jewelry, cell phones, magnets, bio-field devices, keys, etc.

10. The tester should stand slightly to the side of the testee to avoid creating a conflicting energy field by uniting the chakra energy systems in the body.

11. The tester should not look the testee in the eye while muscle testing.

12. Do not cross your arms or legs, or allow the testee to cross theirs. This is most likely to happen if you are testing someone while one of you are sitting.

13. If you have a physical item, such as a bottle of herbs, oils or tincture, that you want to test an individual for, simply have them hold the item in the hand of the arm you are not testing. However, you do not need to physically have whatever you are testing connected to the testee. You can just think of the item, or have the testee think of the item. However, if using only a thought, the person performing the visualization must be able to sustain their focused energy well enough that their mind will not wander during the length of the testing. Energy follows focus.

14. You need to be able to be completely objective about whatever you are testing or the questions you are asking. Once you ask the question, you must hold your mind in a state of absolute silence, or stay focused on the statement or question you are testing with no preconceived notion of

the outcome. If you fail to do this, the results will most likely be skewed.

15. You can self-muscle-test by using the O-ring or thumb/pointer finger technique. Your results should be accurate if you follow rule #15. To test yourself, bring the thumb and pointer finger of your non-dominant hand together, forming an O. Then insert your thumb (of your dominant hand) into the O and connect it with the forefinger of your dominant hand. Ask the question or make the statement, then pull with the thumb of your dominant hand against the area where your finger and thumb from your non-dominant hand meet.

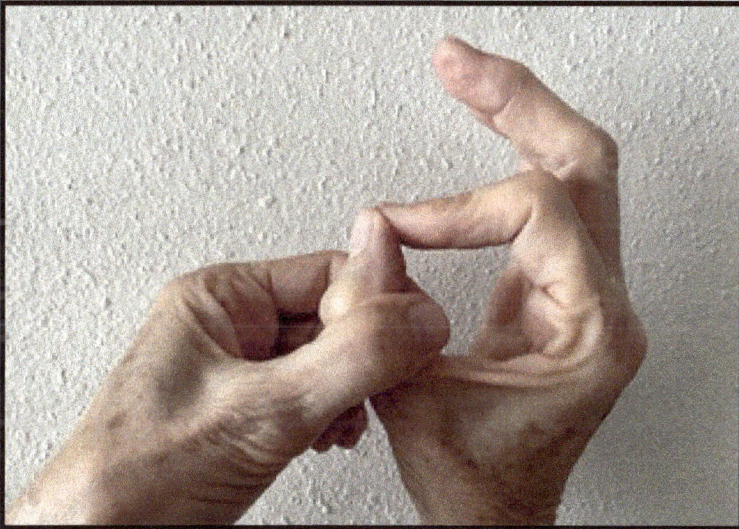

Right-handed

(See next page for Left-handed)

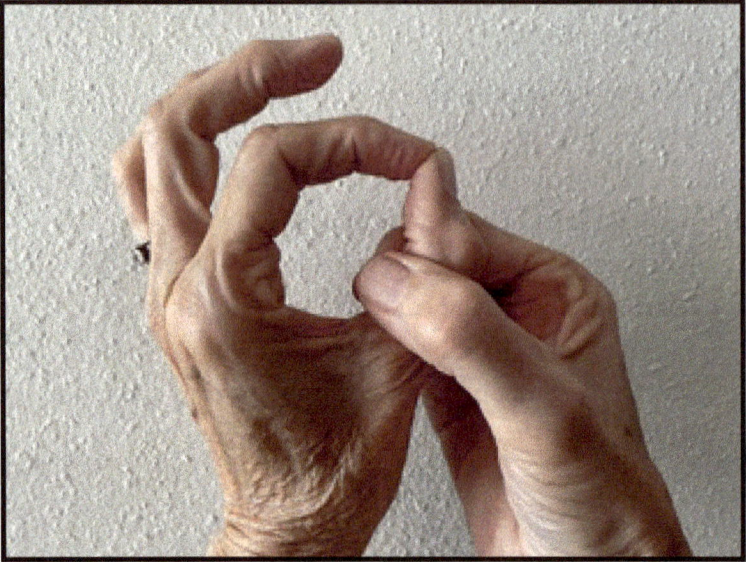

Left-handed

To practice this method, pull gently and firmly using a statement you know to be true such as your name or your age. Then try pulling again with a statement you know is not true. You should not be able to break the O if the statement is true and likewise, you should be able to break the O with a statement that you know is false. Once you have practiced this technique several times with statements you know are true and false and can feel the difference, then try using this technique with something you are unsure about, such as *How many of these herbs should I take right now? Should I take at least one?* (Then test the O), *Should I take at least two?* (Then test the O again.) Using the phrase "at least" as you move up the scale of amounts is very important. After some practice, you will become accurate and not have to guess about a lot of things in the future.

16. Set appropriate parameters with the question. Use a scale of 0-10, or 0-100, etc. For example: *On a scale of 0 to10, how beneficial is this oil for____ (a specific issue)?* or, *On a scale of 0 to 100, if 100 is perfect functioning of the (liver), how well is the (liver) functioning right now? Is it at least 70%, at least 80%?* etc.

17. When assessing emotional issues, have the testee stand or sit with their head straight and eyes open and looking down at a 45-degree angle as you muscle test questions or statements. Emotions are more easily accessed when done this way.

Now you have all the rules that I am aware of for the most accurate muscle testing. However, I have found that people beginning to learn muscle testing can still be very unsure of themselves and doubt their results. So, I have formulated some positive affirmations to help you with those doubts. Say these affirmations to yourself before you muscle test until you feel sure of yourself and your ability:

I affirm that this testing is for my highest good and for the good of all of those around me. Affirming your personal faith increases your accuracy. Modify this in any fashion to personalize it. When you speak it, be sure to put feeling and belief into it.

I trust my intuitive intelligence to clearly communicate my needs. Doubts and skepticism can be normal healthy thoughts. However, their presence during testing muddies the test results. Have the mindset of trusting and you'll get better accuracy.

I set aside my opinion on (name of product, issue, etc.) right now. Opinions are natural, normal, and good things to have. However, they will interfere with accurate test results.

The speed at which I am learning this is ok. I am learning to be more accurate every time I test. Everyone learns at the speed that is right for them. Doing accurate muscle testing takes practice. Don't get discouraged if you find you are unable to do it perfectly right away.

I agree to set aside my experience right now and rely on the success of others. As you learn, there may be times when it feels like muscle testing is not working. However, focusing on the belief that it's not working amplifies that issue. In the meantime, rely on the successes of millions of others who have learned to accurately muscle test.

In the presence of what seems to be contrary evidence, I agree to trust right now. Getting inconsistent results when first learning is normal. However, buying into that evidence and saying to yourself that muscle testing does not work retards your progress. Reconsider how you asked the question. The energy responds to <u>exactly</u> what you say. Maybe there are some words you need to change. Every word can and does make a difference.

Everyone is entitled to their own opinion, so what others think of me is none of my business. Sometimes people judge muscle testing negatively, which is ok. However, letting their opinions affect your feelings hampers your success. Don't burden yourself with their opinions, nor burden them with yours. Allowing others to freely have their opinions frees your mind.

Use a personal mental anchor. Think about a time when you got an intuitive hit - that time when you instinctively knew something that you're sure you didn't know just a second earlier. Put yourself back into that time and place; trust your feelings as you muscle test.

Now that we have covered how to accurately muscle test and how to counter negative thoughts and feelings that could potentially hold you back, it's time to get excited! You can use muscle testing to determine so many things. In fact, the list is endless. But here are some things to consider:

- Recognizing a true statement vs. a false statement that you or someone else is making

- The functioning level of body parts (*On a scale of 1 to 10, what is the functioning level of____? Is it at least a 5, at least a 6*, etc.?)

- What emotional issues are being held onto that are causing this dis-ease?

- *What past events* (whether remembered or not) *are causing this dis-ease? With whom did the past event occur* (mother, father, friend, teacher, etc.)? *Where did the past event occur? At what age did the past event occur?*

- Substances that are good or bad for the body: herbs, vitamins, minerals, foods, homeopathic remedies, essential oils, crystals, gems, laundry detergent, household cleaning products, clothing materials, perfumes, hair dye, makeup, areas to live, etc.

- People that are good or bad for you to be around

- The consciousness levels of people, books, teachings, etc. (*If 1,000 equals Perfect Consciousness, then what is the consciousness level of_____? Is it at least 100?, 200?, etc.*)

- How much and how long you should take herbs, vitamins, etc.

- Which body parts are needing assistance

- Cleanses that need to be done for the body

- Physical therapies that would be good or bad for the body

- Spiritual teachings that would be good or bad for you to pursue

- Future actions you should pursue, including jobs, places to live, people to date, etc. **Please note**: muscle testing for future events is not entirely accurate, especially the further out you try to go into the future. This is because we all have free agency and circumstances can change radically.

Once again, be very careful and precise about how you ask the question. Asking, *Is this herb good for me?* is very vague. Asking *On a scale of 1 - 10, how well will this herb work for my kidney function?* is much more specific. Asking, *Should I move to Arizona?* is vague. Asking, *Should I move to Phoenix, Arizona in January of this next year?* is much more precise. I hope you get the idea.

3

PSYCHONEUROIMMUNOLOGY

A sad soul can be just as lethal as a germ.
~ John Steinbeck

I believe we are eternal beings who came to this planet for the purposes of gaining information and learning lessons that will help us advance spiritually. Many of our life lessons are about setting appropriate boundaries, and of loving correctly and unconditionally. I believe when we are unable to do these things, we are placed in similar events somewhere down the road in our lifetime. This gives us another opportunity to make the proper decisions and develop the mind-set of unconditional love. Hopefully, we get it right. If not, this cycle continues to happen again and again until we do. Some people identify this as karma. If we do not correct our reactions and mind-set, at some point the discordant energy created in our spirits will eventually settle into our bodies giving us a final warning that we need to change our mind-set, our hearts, and how we look at and perceive the world.

Many people have asked me what I mean by unconditional love. A wise counselor once explained it to me this way. There are three people we need to forgive in order to move into unconditional love; our perpetrator, God and ourselves. First, we need to be able forgive the person who wronged us. In order to do this, we need to be able to look at this person as our teacher and ask ourselves, "What did I learn from this person?" Once we understand the lesson we received, we need to thank them (not necessarily to their face) for the lesson they have taught us and then forgive them for what was perceived as their wrong-doing. The second person we need to forgive is God. We often harbor anger at God for putting us into situations that were very difficult and painful. Once again, we need to be able to embrace the lesson that the situation brought us and thank God for putting us in that situation which ultimately left us with greater wisdom and understanding than we had before. Finally, we need to forgive ourselves. If we realize that this life is a university, created to teach us valuable lessons that we will need as eternal beings, then we are able to love and embrace ourselves when we make mistakes. As we become wiser, we will learn to set appropriate boundaries and not allow ourselves to be put in harmful situations or know how to get ourselves out of harmful situations when the need arises.

I have found that love is not only about putting ourselves in another's shoes and helping out, but it is also about setting appropriate boundaries for ourselves because we need to "love our neighbors as ourselves" and not allow others to take advantage of us. There are two major problems with being helpful in situations or in ways that we should not interfere. First, we disrespect ourselves by not setting appropriate boundaries, which places us in a position of allowing our energy to be zapped by others, which in turn creates dis-ease within us. Second, we take away the lessons the other person is supposed to be learning. When we eliminate another person's hardships, they do not have to learn the lessons they should. That life lesson will now have to re-manifest in the future, and usually in a much more intense scenario. Many times, when we think we are being loving by helping someone out of a difficult situation, we are actually just not allowing them to grow from the consequences of their actions. When the act of repenting, learning their lesson, and making restitution are taken away from them, we are actually harming them and creating a worse situation for them in the future.

Let me be clear here. I do not believe all negative situations are karma. Many people are born into this world with difficulties or disabilities, or have difficult situations happen to them because they are either seeking to learn important eternal lessons, or helping those close to them learn important eternal lessons. Therefore, we need to be very thoughtful and prayerful in who we help and how we help. Most of the time the most loving thing to do for people is to help them face their difficulties head on and not just bail them out. We need to help them but we also need to teach them how to rise above their situation while we are helping them.

We were all sent here for a divine purpose. People can also become dis-eased when their life goals are not being met. This usually happens when other people or situations are thwarting them from achieving their deepest inner desires. In childhood, this often occurs from overbearing parents or, as an adult, an overbearing spouse. The person can then become so frustrated and agitated that their bodily processes go awry. This is another case where appropriate boundaries need to be set. We cannot always give ourselves away for what we believe is the benefit of others. There must be an appropriate give and take for everyone.

One of the critical factors I have learned in helping others heal is the need to release the emotional issues tied to the disease. The attached emotional issue must be recognized and addressed if healing is going to be complete. Otherwise, the physical disease will return after the appropriate herbal or nutritional remedy has been stopped. The term used to describe the interactions between the emotional state, nervous system, and immune system is called psychoneuroimmunology. Investigations into these interactions have documented that the mind and attitude play a significant role in the functioning of the immune system (Textbook of Natural Medicine 5th ed., 2020).

Louise Hay brought this science to the forefront in her book, *Heal Your Body and You Can Heal Your Life*, where she made many connections between mental and emotional states and various diseases. There is also a comprehensive desk reference by Michael J Lincoln, Ph.D. titled *Messages from the Body*, which enlightens readers on every possible emotional cause of any ailment troubling people from the top of their heads down to their little toes.

In one of my cases, a young college woman came to me with a case of laryngitis she had been dealing with for a couple of weeks. I put her on an appropriate protocol, but after another three weeks it was still unresolved. At this point we decided to muscle test to find out what had happened on an emotional level to cause the issue. Muscle testing revealed that a college professor had criticized her on an assignment and had embarrassed her in class. She ranted about it in her mind for a time, never talked to the professor, and then totally forgot the situation. But even though she had buried the incident and no longer remembered it, her psyche had not forgotten. The laryngitis cleared within a couple of days once we brought the situation back to her memory and discussed the appropriate actions to take if it ever happened again.

In a more dramatic case, I was working with a 16-year-old young man who had been diagnosed with Asperger's syndrome. I will call him Joey. I had been treating Joey for about six months for various physical issues we were able to get resolved. During one of the sessions, I explained to his mother that we could also look into emotional issues that could be holding back his development. The L.I.F.E. quantum biofeedback system I use in my practice is able to go into emotional issues a person is still dealing with and give hints of the situation that might have caused the problem from the past. It provides the age, emotional conflict, situation, and type of person involved in the life conflict. I felt that by exploring these various issues, he might progress in his social life. The mother was extremely interested and, with his permission, we decided to proceed. Before we began the session, the young man would barely make eye contact, had no interest in developing meaningful relationships with friends or girlfriends, and had no interest in getting a driver's license or a job.

Joey started coming for L.I.F.E. sessions monthly. We had him relax during the session while the L.I.F.E. system scanned his energy field and brought up hints pertaining to unresolved emotional issues. As I talked to him, he could hardly remember any of these situations, but his mother remembered practically all of them. As the L.I.F.E. system treats the emotional issues by sending energy frequencies to help clear them, it also gives a reading as to how well the situation is being resolved. In most of the situations we would see very little response when I would first apply the healing frequencies. But when his mother helped him remember the situation that he had forgotten, the L.I.F.E. system would quickly begin to show numbers indicating that the unresolved issues were being cleared.

The emotional transformation that took place in this young man was truly amazing. Over the next nine months, Joey began to make eye contact, got a job and a driving license, made a couple of friends, and even had a blossoming relationship with a girl he proudly called his girlfriend. Buried emotional issues he was unable to deal with appropriately as a child had been holding back his adulthood. It was incredibly heartwarming to watch!

Another great book to add to your reading list is Karol K. Truman's, *Feelings Buried Alive Never Die*. We never really get rid of emotional issues until they are confronted and resolved. They just get buried deep in the cellular memory of our bodies and cause dis-ease. In order to affect complete and permanent healing, we cannot forget to heal ourselves emotionally as well as physically.

***

Throughout the following chapters, I will be addressing some emotional root causes of dis-ease as we talk about cleansing the various organ systems of the body. I will be lightly touching on the science of psychoneuroimmunology there. For a much more comprehensive view of this connection, please refer to one of the books mentioned in the references.

4

GENERAL NUTRITION

Let food be thy medicine and medicine be thy food.
~ Hippocrates

Before we get into cleansing, let's talk about the importance of nutrition. All of the cells in the body need the proper nutrients and hydration to perform their functions. Vitamins, minerals, amino acids, essential fatty acids, and antioxidants are all critical nutrients.

It would be wonderful if we could feel confident that our foods are supplying all of our nutritional needs. Unfortunately, in our day and age, our foods are not able to supply these things for us. Food is usually picked long before it is ripened, which does not allow the proper amount of nutrients to be formed in the plant. Our foods have also been corrupted by chemical fertilizers and pesticides, not to mention being genetically modified, making most nutrients totally unavailable. On top of that, a lot of people order from a fast-food menu, which is almost completely devoid of any kind of nutritional content. In addition to not providing the nutrients we need, many of the things we consume are extremely damaging to our bodies. While it is abundantly clear that diets in the United States, as well as many developed countries, include an overabundance of calories. A growing body of evidence shows that even though we are eating more, we are also obtaining fewer of the essential nutrients vital for optimal health.

Over-processed, calorie-rich, nutrient-poor food choices threaten to make us fat even as our bodies are deprived of critical essential nutrients. The American Medical Association acknowledges the importance of taking nutritional supplements, admitting that while "the clinical syndromes of vitamin deficiencies are unusual in Western societies, suboptimal vitamin status is not." (Journal of the American Medical Association, June 19, 2002).

Unfortunately, this situation cannot be solved by merely taking a bunch of vitamin supplements. For instance, some nutritional supplement manufacturers add many times the necessary amount of synthetic vitamins and minerals to their products to persuade consumers that "more is better." In reality, more does not always offer additional benefits and may simply be more expensive, as well as toxic to the body. Yes, an overabundance of nutrients can actually create a toxic condition. When this happens, the liver and kidneys will simply eliminate the nutrients as quickly as possible, still leaving the cells deprived. This approach also creates very expensive urine since the body simply flushes the excess out of the body. Sometimes the vitamin supplement simply passes through the digestive system completely undissolved.

When I was doing research during my doctoral program, I came across a very interesting story by a researcher who was studying the absorbency of various vitamins. One of the ways he did this was by going to port-a-potty dump sites and looking to see what was left in the remains. At one dump site, he noticed a pile of white pills on the ground. As he examined them more closely, he discovered they were popular vitamins designed specifically for adults aged 50 and older. He could tell what they were because the label was still visible on the pill. This particular brand is very popular with older citizens because it is one of the least expensive vitamin options that claims to be "specifically formulated to meet the nutritional needs of adults 50 years of age and over." The problem is that, around the age of 50, our hydrochloric acid and other digestive enzymes begin to drop off, sometimes significantly. These pills are coated with a substance that makes them nearly impossible for any body, especially an older one, to absorb.

Choosing a balanced vitamin/mineral supplement with a comprehensive array of whole-food vitamins and minerals, along with essential fatty acids and antioxidants, is critical to optimal health. For those over the age of 50, I also recommend a good, balanced digestive enzyme.

We also need a clean supply of uncontaminated drinking water. Chlorine and fluoride are the two most common toxic chemicals in tap water. But that is not all; other harmful substances such as herbicides, lead, mercury, nitrates, pharmaceuticals, pesticides, and chemical fertilizers can also be in our tap water. A lot of people will go to the store and spend a lot of money buying water in disposable plastic bottles, thinking that will solve the problem. Unfortunately, what you are drinking instead is a lot of plastic micro-particles. One liter of bottled water can contain hundreds of thousands of plastic particles and polyfluoroalkyl substances, (PFAS), or forever chemicals. They are called "forever" because they do not break down in the environment, nor in the human body. Having even a small amount of these in your body can lead to cancer.

This is especially true with women and breast cancer, as an abundance of nano plastics are being found in and around cancerous breast tissue.

Returning to the fluoride issue, this substance is supposedly added to our water in order to strengthen our teeth. Originally, fluoride was added to municipal water supplies as a way to dispose of a by-product of the aluminum mining industry. Even though the amount added to our drinking water is considered safe by the Environmental Protection Agency (EPA), the higher-than-normal amounts consumed eventually accumulate in our bodies, causing liver and kidney issues while calcifying the pineal gland. A calcified pineal gland causes insomnia, migraines, premature aging and other neurodegenerative diseases such as Alzheimer's Disease.

The pineal gland is a small, pea-shaped endocrine gland located deep in the center of the brain, between the two hemispheres. It plays a crucial role in regulating biological rhythms, primarily by producing and regulating hormones, especially melatonin, which influences sleep-wake cycles. It is often referred to as the "third eye" and some philosophical traditions associate it with spiritual awakening.

The best way to get clean drinking water is to buy a good water filtration system that removes all of these harmful chemicals. We recommend the Berkey gravity water filtration system which is relatively inexpensive and removes 99.9% of everything harmful in your water. Berkey systems are used in disaster areas by the Red Cross and United Way, since they can be used to produce pure drinking water from a polluted river or stream. It is a portable unit that sits on your counter, does not require any power source, and does not use more water during filtration than it produces. You simply fill the container with regular tap water from your faucet and it will drip through the filters, providing clean drinking water out of the spigot on the bottom of the unit. The filters last for thousands of gallons by easily cleaning them off when filtration begins to run slowly. Since no power source is needed, the Berkey system is an excellent item to have in case of emergency situations. Berkey also sells portable water bottles you can take with you when you travel, eliminating the need for endless purchases of plastic-bottled water. (See jamesjmaguire.com to order this product.)

Once we have given the body the nutritional support and proper hydration that it needs, we can move on to cleaning out the debris using some well-known researched herbs and essential oils.

5

HERBS AND TINCTURES

*And may we ever have gratitude in our hearts that the
great Creator in all His glory has placed the herbs in
the field for our healing.*
~ Edward Bach

Herbs are superfoods. Herbs help people improve their health
naturally. Herbs are not new. They have been used since people
began eating, long before there were doctors or scientists.
Herbs were effective thousands of years ago, and they still work
today. In the beginning, a lot of intuition, trial, and error were
used in choosing the appropriate herbs for a particular ailment.
After all those years of experimenting, we now have a long list
of herbs and their various uses that is well-documented by
anecdotal and scientific evidence.

Luckily, if you only take a small amount of the wrong herb,
the body will simply eliminate it and you will have very few, if
any, side effects. Oftentimes, an herb will taste nasty to
someone when they don't need it, but will taste delicious when
they do need it.

Most of today's pharmaceutical medicines have been
derived from herbal remedies. Prescription drugs are
concentrates, fractionated from the active constituents in herbs
or created synthetically. The difference is the medications do
not contain the original buffers that the plant has. When the

active ingredients are separated from the buffers naturally found in the plants, all kinds of side-effects can occur. This creates a cascade of effects that begins with just one little medication that is prescribed to treat an ailment. But that drug causes side-effects, so new drugs are prescribed for those. But they have side-effects as well, so they require even more drugs. Soon, the patient is finding themselves overwhelmed by the cost and the effort of dealing with all these innocent little pills. So much pain, suffering, money, and effort would be saved if people had the knowledge that would allow them to go back to using the natural remedies from which these drugs were derived. This does not even begin to address any psychological effects that come from having to take so many medications.

It has been said that everyone has their own unique herb that suits them best and will heal and strengthen them most of the time. I wish you the best of luck in exploring the use of herbal plants and finding your unique gift from the Creator.

6

ESSENTIAL OILS

If you believe in Aromatherapy... it works!
If you don't believe in Aromatherapy... it works!
~ Cristina Proano-Carrion

Essential oils are volatile liquids, meaning they will evaporate quickly at room temperature. They are distilled from the barks, leaves, flowers, fruits, and roots of plants. They have been used for thousands of years, as recorded in Egyptian and Chinese manuscripts. They have also been found in the ink of cave paintings. Rene-Maurice Gattefosse was a French chemist, born in 1881, who repopularized essential oils. He is credited with coining the term aromatherapy and is known as the Father of Aromatherapy.

Although aromatherapy lost its popularity with the rise of modern drugs, it went through a recent resurgence, beginning with Robert Tisserand. Tisserand searched for a copy of Gattefosse's book, *Gattefosse's Aromatherapy* for 20 years. He was thrilled when he was able to find it, edit it, and republish it under the original title. In 1974, Tisserand founded the first school for aromatherapy, Tisserand Aromatherapy in the UK, and is credited with making information about the therapeutic uses of essential oils widely available to the global public.

One of the factors determining the purity, potency, and therapeutic value of essential oils is their chemical makeup, or constituents. These can be influenced by several things, including: the part of the plant used to distill the oil, the condition of the soil, the type of fertilizer (organic or chemical), the geographic region, the climate, the altitude, the harvest season, and the method of extraction. Obtaining an essential oil that has been grown, harvested, and distilled properly to make it of the highest therapeutic value can be costly. If you plan on using them for therapeutic purposes, you want to make sure the oils are 100% therapeutic grade. Synthetic oils are easily found and inexpensive, but they are not safe for therapeutic use. At best, they will not work at all; at worst, they will cause you more harm than good.

Essential oils embody the regenerating, protective, and immune-strengthening properties of plants. A good therapeutic essential oil has the ability to affect every cell of your body within 20 minutes. Many essential oils have antibacterial, anti-fungal, anti-infectious, antimicrobial, anti-tumor, anti-parasitic, antiviral, and antiseptic properties. Essential oils are basically what a plant uses to protect itself, and these same oils can help protect us.

Keep in mind that essential oils are highly concentrated. They can be used topically by applying them directly to the affected area to help soft tissues through massage, reflexology, compresses and baths. They can be applied on the wrist or arch of the foot near blood vessels in order to get the oils into the bloodstream and systemically throughout the body. Caution is needed with many essential oils, especially the "hot" ones such as cinnamon, oregano, or black pepper. It is best to mix hotter oils with a carrier oil, such as coconut oil, to eliminate sensitivity of the skin. All essential oils should be diluted for use with small children or pets.

Essential oils can be used aromatically by diffusing them, directly inhaling them from the bottle, inhaling from a drop on a cloth or tissue, putting some on a cotton ball in front of a fan or vent, or using them as perfume or cologne.

Only pure therapeutic grade essential oils should be used internally and with caution. The liver and kidneys can become overwhelmed with the amount of essential oils being used, causing undue stress. Drinking essential oils in water continuously can negatively affect the delicate lining of the esophagus over time. You can also put essential oils in capsules, use them in cooking, or as a vaginal or rectal insertion.

Like herbs, essential oils come from plants. They are more potent in many ways than herbal remedies, but do not contain the vitamins and other nutrients of herbs. Essential oils may cause more negative skin reactions and heightened sensitivities than herbs. Both essential oils and herbs are wonderful remedies from nature, and you will need to experiment to find a balance in using them together.

7

BODY SYSTEMS

Take care of your body. It's the only place you have to live.
~ Jim Rohn

In order to understand how to systematically cleanse your body, you need to understand your body's different biological systems. Science has divided the body into 11 systems. These different systems each have their own unique structure and function. They include:

1. Digestive: mouth, esophagus, stomach, small intestine, colon

2. Cardiovascular: heart, arteries and veins

3. Hepatic: liver, gallbladder, bile duct

4. Lymphatic/Immune: lymph glands, tonsils, thymus, spleen

5. Renal or Urinary: kidneys, ureters, bladder

6. Integumentary: skin, hair, nails, sweat glands

7. Respiratory: lungs, trachea

8. Musculoskeletal: muscles and bones

9. Endocrine: hormones

10. Nervous: central and peripheral nerves

11. Reproductive: sex organs

Some of these body systems can be specifically cleansed but others will be cleansed when we eliminate parasites, yeast and chemicals/heavy metals. I have learned a specific order for doing these cleanses in order to prevent my clients from having uncomfortable reactions during the process.

This is the proper order for cleansing.

1. Colon cleanse

2. Circulatory cleanse

3. Liver/Gallbladder cleanse

4. Kidney cleanse

5. Lymphatic cleanse

6. Parasite cleanse

7. Yeast cleanse

8. Environmental/Heavy metal cleanse

***

The last three cleanses get rid of unwanted "critters", man-made chemicals, and heavy metals. These things will accumulate in the body when they have sufficient food and when there are poor detoxification and elimination channels. I also believe they are the root causes of many, if not all, cancers, so it is extremely important to keep them out of the body.

Years of experience have taught me that when I am attempting to help clients cleanse their bodies, daily lifestyle must be considered. People still have their lives to live while cleansing and if a program becomes too harsh, people are much more likely to abandon it. So be careful in trying to cleanse too much at once if you do not want a healing crisis on your hands. For the most part, do the cleanses in the order they are listed. However, many healthy people can usually combine the cleansing of the colon with the circulatory cleanse. They can also usually combine the liver/gallbladder cleanse with the kidney cleanse. The lymphatic system and the parasite cleanse can work together if the person does not already have a lot of mucus or swollen lymph nodes. Often, the yeast cleanse and the heavy metal detox can be done together. Consider the health and strength of the person cleansing. If they are healthy and strong, combining cleanses can speed up the process. However, if they are weak and sickly, it is best to do the cleanses separately. If you are not doing muscle testing to determine the length of the cleanse, then just stay with the single cleanse or combination of cleanses for at least a month before going to the next one.

In the following chapters, I will be discussing the cleansing process, herbs, and essential oils that can be beneficial along with dietary recommendations to use while you are doing the cleanses. Please, keep in mind, I am only giving a sampling of the products that can be helpful. It is not my intention to give a complete list of all of the products that can be used for various issues. There are many other excellent books that have already addressed this. My main intent is to provide the cleansing process and the proper order to follow for the best results. At the back of this book under the title RESOURCES you will find extremely beneficial information to refer to along your journey.

I also want to add a **CAUTIONARY NOTE**: If you are very weak, are on a lot of medications, or are on medications for psychosis, your heart, or other life-threatening illnesses, please consult your doctor before doing these cleanses. Some of the cleanses will pull medications out of your system. There may also be other situations where doing these cleanses, or using certain herbs or essential oils, are contraindicated. Be safe!

PART 2
CLEANSING
AND
SUPPORTING

8

THE COLON

All disease begins in the gut.
~ Hippocrates

The digestive system includes the mouth, esophagus, stomach, small intestines, and colon. These organs break down the carbohydrates we consume into sugars, and the proteins into amino acids. They also extract the vitamins, minerals, sugars, and fats from our food that the body needs for energy, growth, and repair.

When food is chewed, saliva in the mouth breaks down carbohydrates into sugars. It is important to chew food thoroughly so this process can occur. Food should feel very liquidy when you swallow it. Otherwise, undigested food can get stuck in the esophagus, and undigested carbohydrates can cause gas and bloating. Many digestive health concerns can be alleviated by this practice alone.

Once food is swallowed, it goes down the esophagus through the lower esophageal sphincter (LES) and enters the stomach. If the LES doesn't close properly, stomach contents and acid can move back up into the esophagus causing burning and a condition called Gastroesophageal reflux or GERD, commonly known as heartburn. When food reaches the stomach, the stomach squeezes and churns the food to break it down while secreting gastric juices, mucus, pepsin, and hydrochloric acid (HCL). Pepsin, along with HCL, are the digestive enzymes that break proteins into amino acids. Mucus protects the stomach lining from being harmed by the powerful acids. Stomach acids also destroy bacteria, parasites, and other dangerous organisms.

From the stomach, food travels into the small intestine. Here food is broken down and nutrients are absorbed. Ninety percent of nutrients are absorbed in the small intestine, including vitamins, minerals, carbohydrates, fats, proteins, and electrolytes or minerals. Undigested food is sent to the colon for further absorption of water, then undigested food, fiber, and dead bacteria are expelled.

A sticky, tar-like mucus can accumulate in our intestines throughout our life when we eat a lot of soft foods devoid of their natural fibers. This tar-like substance clings to the bowel wall, causing auto-intoxication, where toxins are not eliminated but reabsorbed back into the bloodstream.

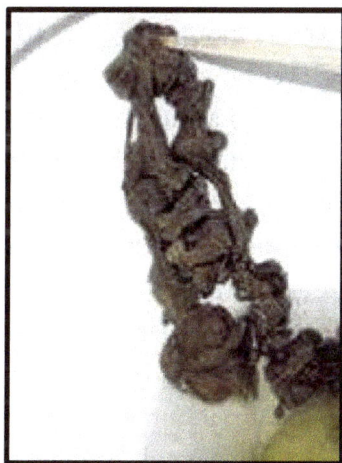

This is a picture of fecal tar or mucoid plaque that has been eliminated during a colonic cleanse.

The most common symptom people experience when they need a colon cleanse is sluggish elimination. However, sometimes it's not sluggish elimination that is the problem — sometimes it is watery stools. This can happen because the colon is irritated by something and the colon is trying to increase its output to get rid of it. We may also experience gas or bloating due to stuck undigested food, rectal itching due to parasites, or abdominal pain and foul-smelling feces due to an imbalance between good and bad intestinal bacteria. We may also see undigested food and mucus in the stool. Sluggish elimination and constipation can be a result of not drinking enough water, a sedentary lifestyle, a lack of exercise, a sluggish thyroid, not having enough hydrochloric acid (HCL) in the stomach, not receiving enough bile from the liver and gallbladder, kidney stones, or not enough fiber in the diet.

To cleanse and rebuild the colon, first, drink more water. Dehydration is a common cause of constipation. When the body is dehydrated, it absorbs more water from the stools, making them harder and more difficult to pass. There is a great deal of controversy over how much a person should drink in a day. I would recommend that you watch for these symptoms to tell if you are dehydrated: constipation; dry mouth, lips, or tongue; dark yellow, strong-smelling urine; feeling thirsty; feeling lightheaded; urinating less than usual; feeling tired; having dark circles under the eyes, skin that is more wrinkled, or fingertips that are cracking. If you are dehydrated, it is not helpful to drink a large amount of water all at once. You will most likely pee it out in about 20 minutes and it will not hydrate you. It is also not helpful to drink a lot of water daily without replenishing electrolytes or minerals. You can do this by dissolving a pinch of sea salt or Himalayan salt in your water or under your tongue. Eating fruits is a great way to hydrate. They contain a lot of water and minerals combined. Otherwise, drinking a small amount of water throughout the day is the most helpful to resolve dehydration.

Bentonite clay and psyllium hulls work wonderfully for a colon cleanse, but should not be taken on a daily basis. Bentonite clay is a natural clay derived from volcanic ash and is very absorbent. The tar-like mucus that has accumulated in your colon will stick to the clay because of an opposite ionic charge, which then pulls it away from the colon and allows it to be eliminated. Bentonite not only helps relieve constipation but also diarrhea because it can neutralize and absorb toxins in the intestinal tract. Another added benefit is that parasites are unable to reproduce in the presence of bentonite clay.

Psyllium becomes gelatinous when soaked in water. It acts as a colon "broom", cleansing the intestinal walls and absorbing toxins. If you take psyllium, be sure to take it with a full glass of water. If you do not drink enough water when you take this fiber, it will be constipating. Also be mindful that it will absorb fat in foods, which is helpful if you are trying to lose weight, but it will also absorb your beneficial omega fatty acids. So it is a good idea to take your psyllium at a different time than your omegas. For example, take your Omega fatty acids with breakfast and take the psyllium hulls at night. Psyllium hulls can also help with weight loss, support lower cholesterol levels, relieve hemorrhoids and absorb toxins produced by Candida. It's also very beneficial at calming Irritable Bowel Syndrome (IBS).

If psyllium is not your friend because it causes gas and bloating, you can also take eight to ten capsules of alfalfa or get a fiber that does not include psyllium.

Aloe Vera is also an excellent choice for bowel issues. The use of Aloe Vera dates back over 4,000 years. The gel is taken from the inner part of the plant. *Aloe Vera* cools inflammation and enhances the immune system. It is anti-inflammatory, antibacterial, and antiviral. *Aloe Vera* is used widely for the treatment of inflammatory bowel disease, peptic ulcers, diabetes, high cholesterol, and high triglyceride levels. You can drink ½ cup of *Aloe Vera* juice in the morning and at night.

Cascara Sagrada comes from the bark of a tree and is one of the most wonderful bowel cleansers found in nature. In Spanish the name means Sacred Bark. Animals in the wild nibble away at this to help them stay regular. If using capsules, start with just two with dinner and work your way up if you need to use more in order to produce two to three bowel movements daily. Although it is not recommended for continual use, it can be used frequently. If chronic constipation is an issue, increase good probiotics and do a liver and gallbladder cleanse to get more bile flowing in order to stimulate the intestines to move.

***

Probiotics are critical to the health of the colon. The good bacteria in the gut make vitamins B1, B9, B12 and K. It also produces over 90% of the body's serotonin, which affects mood, sleep, appetite, and pain sensitivity. Good gut bacteria, also called the intestinal biome, protects the interior lining of the intestines and protects against parasites and yeast. It is important to choose a probiotic capsule that contains several different types of good bacteria so they will compete with each other, which keeps them healthy.

A small sampling of probiotics and their functions include:

- *Lactobacillus* helps digest lactose found in dairy products.

- *Bifidobacterium* is found in small children and in the uterine area of women.

- *Saccharomyces Boulardii* is a yeast bacterium that helps fight off harmful micro-organisms.

- *Lactobacillus Reuteri* is anti-microbial and produces vitamin B-12.

- *Bifidobacterium Longum* helps break down food and absorb nutrients.

- *Lactobacillus Plantarum*, *Lactobacillus Brevis*, and *Bifidobacterium Brevis* all help produce serotonin in the gut.

Some probiotics may also contain fructooligosaccharides (pronounced frook-tow-uh-li-guh-sa-kr-idez) or FOS, which is a prebiotic fiber that feeds beneficial bacteria until they get established. It is critical that the probiotics have a coating on the capsule that keeps it from opening in the stomach. This will be advertised as enteric coated, protected from stomach acid, time released, or double encapsulated. Since it is the stomach acid's job to break down protein, it will also destroy probiotics which are protein. Approximately 85% of an unprotected probiotic formula will be destroyed in the stomach before it ever gets to the intestines. You will not only end up wasting a lot of money but you may also get an upset stomach and diarrhea. It is better to pay a little extra for the protective coating.

***

Essential oils that can be helpful to the intestinal tract include:

- Peppermint Oil (*Mentha x piperita*) is great to use when your belly feels queasy or bloated. Peppermint has been found to relax the muscles in the digestive system to offer soothing relief.

- Ginger Oil (*Zingiber Officinale*) helps soothe queasiness as well as soothing other sore, achy issues. Ginger oil is hot and spicy, so make sure to dilute.

- Anise Oil (*Pimpinella Anisum*) and fennel (*Foeniculum Vulgare*) have powerful calming and spasm reducing components. Their scent is very similar to licorice and can also help reduce queasiness and gas. <u>DO NOT USE it if you have a bleeding disorder or take anticoagulant medication.</u>

- Cardamom Oil (*Elettaria Cardamomum*) is one of the most popular traditional oils for soothing stomach spasms. It promotes the secretion of digestive juices and enzymes to ease digestive upset and bloating.

- Black Pepper (*Piper Nigrum*) is very stimulating to the digestive tract and colon.

In general, good nutrition that keeps the colon cleansed and healthy includes foods such as: whole fruits, vegetables that are raw or lightly steamed, nuts and seeds, beans, lentils, and whole grains, such as brown or wild rice, quinoa, and whole wheat or sprouted grain breads. Prunes and figs are great natural laxatives. The roughage or fiber in these foods helps scrape the walls of the intestines to help keep mucoid plaque from building up. Soft, overly processed foods, such as non-fibrous white breads, rolls, cookies, white rice, and potatoes, are more likely to become impacted against the intestinal walls. Once impacted, they create mucoid plaque or hardened fecal matter where parasites, yeast and bacteria can breed. It is also helpful to follow a low-fat diet and eliminate fried foods.

***

From Psychoneuroimmunology, we learn there is a mind-body connection with the colon. People with colon issues tend to be closed-minded and will not let go of the past. They may be overly conscientious, analytical, hypersensitive, and insecure. They see everything as dangerous and double-dealing. They most likely feel unappreciated and rushed, and are desperate for affection. They can also be overly critical and frequently find fault with other people.

***

Some great positive affirmations for colon health:

- *I easily release that which I no longer need.*

- *I love and approve of myself. I am safe.*

- *I trust the process of life.*

- *Out with the old; in with the new.*
- *The past is over and I am free.*

As we cleanse our emotions, become more confident, let go of the past, and move forward in love for our fellow beings and ourselves, we can support our body systems so they can function properly. It will also work the other way around. Cleansing our body systems will affect how we view our world and others, hopefully bringing us into greater peace and harmony.

9

THE CIRCULATORY SYSTEM

It is only with the heart that one can see rightly;
what is essential is invisible to the eye.
- Antoine de Saint-Exupéry

The next cleanse, in order of priority, is the cardiovascular system. The reason we do it next is that the cleanses for other organ systems, Candida/yeast, or parasites dumps a lot of mucus and debris into the lymphatic system, where it is then dumped into the cardiovascular system for delivery to the liver and then intestines, where it is finally eliminated. If the cardiovascular system is already congested, these cleanses could ultimately increase congestion, which in turn could cause other health issues, such as high blood pressure.

I discovered this the hard way when I did a parasite cleanse on a young lady without checking to see if her arteries and other organ systems were clear. We were both attending a party and the host invited me to demonstrate muscle testing. I tested this lady, who was a close friend, but not a current client. The muscle testing indicated that she needed a parasite cleanse. We then tested further for which herbs would work best and how much of each to take. After the party, she secured the products from the local health food store and started the cleanse. She called me after about seven days into the cleanse to tell me that she had just been to the emergency room the night before with extremely high blood pressure and a bloody nose that would not stop until they cauterized it. She had not been aware of any high blood pressure issues before that time. She asked me if the parasite cleanse could have caused the problem. Initially, I told her no. But after I thought about it for a while, I wondered if it did. Since we did the muscle testing at the party, I had not checked her to see if she needed any of the other cleanses. I invited her to see me so I could do more muscle testing. Sure enough, her arteries and her liver were congested. The cleanse had dumped mucus into the bloodstream, creating more congestion in the arteries and liver, causing her blood pressure to spike.

The circulatory system consists of the heart, arteries, veins, and capillaries. Oxygen-rich blood leaves the left side of the heart and enters the largest artery, called the aorta. The aorta branches into smaller arteries, which then branch into even smaller vessels. The smallest vessels are called capillaries. It is here that the blood gives its nutrients and oxygen to the cells and takes in carbon dioxide, water, and waste. Waste is removed from the bloodstream by the kidneys, liver, spleen and lungs. Blood not only transports oxygen, but also nutrients, hormones, antibodies, and many other substances the body needs. It is essentially like the highway transportation system of the body. Blood also helps maintain our body temperature, our pH balance, and our electrolyte, or mineral, balance.

Heart disease is the number one killer in America today. In the United States, someone has a heart attack every thirty-four seconds. It is very easy to be unaware you have a problem because you cannot really feel its effects until it's too late. That is why it is often called the "silent killer."

Most heart attacks occur from a buildup of low-density lipoproteins (LDL), or bad cholesterol, in the veins. However, a heart attack can also occur if the arteries that feed the heart are weak or collapsing. This can occur either from free radical damage from chemical toxins, from excess insulin, or from glucose, which pits and corrodes arterial walls. This is why diabetes has been linked to heart disease. High density lipoproteins (HDL) help keep LDL from building up plaque in the arteries, but do not prevent veins from collapsing.

Excess homocysteine and C-reactive proteins are indicators of inflammation in the veins, which causes plaque build-up, heart disease, and weakened blood vessels. Recent research has shown that inflammation is often responsible for the blockages that cause heart attacks, strokes, and peripheral vascular disease in the feet and legs. Low levels of vitamins B6, B12, and Folic acid have been directly linked to high levels of homocysteine.

Free radicals from chemical toxins and natural bodily processes pit and corrode arterial walls, making them weak — possibly to the point of collapse. Free radicals also cause cholesterol to build up in the veins and arteries. Dr. Denham Harmon became famous for having discovered free radicals or, more accurately, for developing the "free radical concept of aging."

Free radicals are unstable molecules that have an odd number of electrons in their outer ring. Electrons prefer to have even pairs, so when a free radical is floating around in your bloodstream, it will steal an electron out of the cell walls of the veins and arteries. This causes oxidative stress, like rust on a bumper, which will damage or destroy healthy, functioning cells. This stress will go on to speed up the aging process by compromising cellular DNA and other critical cell structures. Some free radicals are a natural, toxic by-product of breathing and of metabolizing food. Free radicals also come from other sources, such as: pollution, chemicals found in pesticides, smoking, sun exposure, and exposure to radiation. Although the body produces antioxidants and also receives antioxidants by eating foods that contain vitamin C, E and beta-carotene, the number of free radicals from inside and outside sources can push oxidative stress beyond what the body can safely handle.

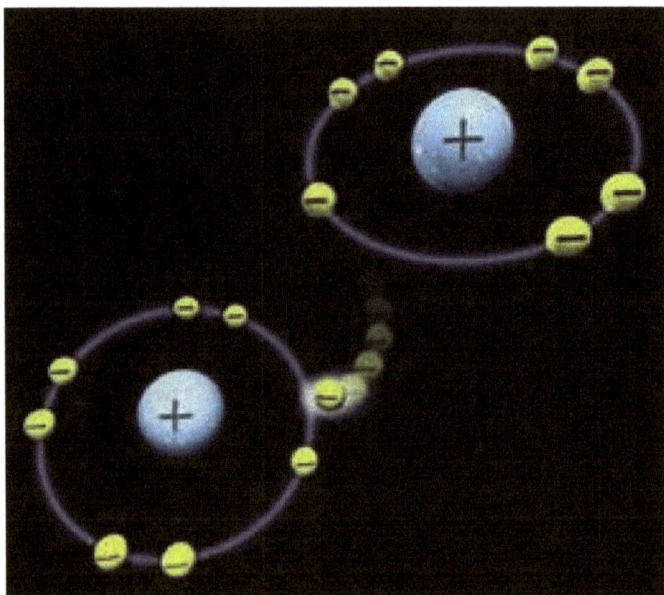

This is a free radical stealing an electron.

This nipping away of the cells in your veins and arteries is like a cut on the surface of your skin. When your skin gets cut, the damaged cells senses danger, become inflamed and a scab develops to protect the area. Similar to how your skin creates a scab to protect damaged cells, cholesterol travels inside of your veins and covers damaged areas. Cholesterol is a sticky substance, so as more cholesterol flows through the veins, it bumps into the cholesterol scab and becomes stuck as well, creating more layers of plaque.

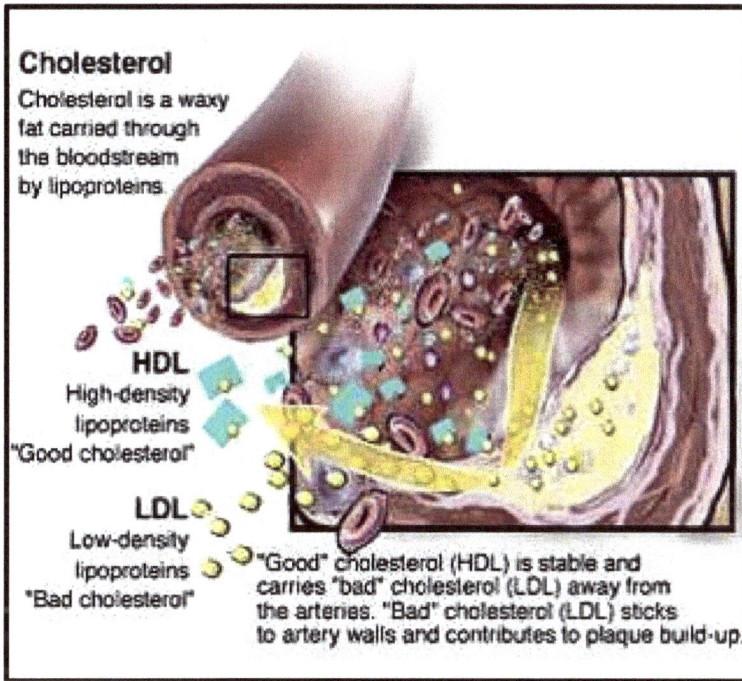

Cholesterol

Cholesterol is a waxy fat carried through the bloodstream by lipoproteins.

HDL
High-density lipoproteins
"Good cholesterol"

LDL
Low-density lipoproteins
"Bad cholesterol"

"Good" cholesterol (HDL) is stable and carries "bad" cholesterol (LDL) away from the arteries. "Bad" cholesterol (LDL) sticks to artery walls and contributes to plaque build-up.

In this picture, we see the yellow plaque build-up. HDL's responsibility is to clean up the plaque from sticky cholesterol. Good fats that form HDLs are found in fatty fish or fish oil, avocado oil, nuts and seeds, olive oil, and flaxseed oil.

Antioxidants have a lot of extra electrons and happily give them to free radicals, protecting the cells of your body from becoming damaged. CoQ10 is a wonderful antioxidant for the heart and arteries. Foods high in antioxidants are beans, berries, apples, spinach, green tea, and dark chocolate. Don't you just love the last one! When you get used to the taste of a good dark chocolate, you will never go back to eating milk chocolate again!

***

A few herbs that are very helpful for the cardiovascular system include:

- Butcher's Broom (*Ruscus Aculeatus*) helps tighten and strengthen the walls of blood vessels.

- Hawthorn berries (*Crataegus*) help improve the tone of the cardiac muscle and heart valves.

- Cayenne or capsicum (*Capsicum Annuum*), chickweed (*Stellaria Media*), and Maidenhair tree (*Ginkgo Biloba*) are excellent at helping reduce plaque buildup.

- Mega Chel (NSP) is an amazing product! I have used this hundreds of times with clients. It has been observed by medical testing that, over several months, Mega Chel can effectively support clean and healthy arteries.

***

Essential oils that can be helpful for heart and circulation include:

- Holy Basil (*Ocimum Basilicum*) is shown to lower bad cholesterol levels. It has antioxidant properties that can help alleviate damage to the arteries, by reducing plaque buildup.

- Cassia (*Cassia Auriculata*) is shown to lower blood glucose levels. When blood sugar levels are high, more plaque builds up on the arterial walls. It was also demonstrated to be more effective than lavender at reducing high blood pressure.

- Ginger (*Zingiber Officinale*) is shown to reduce cholesterol and inhibit oxidation of arterial walls.

- Lemon (*Citrus Limon*) can help remove plaque in the bloodstream and lower blood pressure.

- Rosemary (*Salvia Rosmarinus*) can be used internally or topically to bring cholesterol back into balance.

***

Nutrition for healthy arteries includes foods such as: fruits and vegetables, lean meats, fish high in Omega 3 fatty acids, and whole grains such as oatmeal and brown rice. Use plant-based oils such as: olive oil or avocado oil. Cherries contain antioxidants that protect blood vessels and prevent inflammation. Cinnamon improves blood flow, widens blood vessels and can lower bad cholesterol. Finally, dark chocolate is rich in polyphenols and can help decrease inflammation in the arteries.

Want to increase your chances of heart disease? Eat foods high in saturated fats, such as: fried foods, French fries, potato chips, fatty meats, bacon, hot dogs, salami, and butter. Don't forget to include foods that contain added sugars, like those found in: sodas, sweets, cookies, cakes, and alcohol. These foods should be especially avoided during this cleanse.

***

Psychoneuroimmunology indicates the mind-body connection for those who have heart and artery disease is that of a broken heart. They typically have suppressed grief and pain, and may often feel like a failure who is unworthy or undeserving of love. They usually have high anxiety and work furiously. They may be unable to express emotions in positive ways and may become heartless, developing a hardening of the heart and attitudes that is reflected in the physical hardening of their arteries.

***

Some beautiful affirmations for the heart:

- *God is fully supporting me.*

- *I choose to see life with love.*

- *I choose to love life.*

- *I am bringing joy back into my life.*

- *Every beat of my heart brings more joy.*

10

THE LIVER AND GALLBLADDER

Is life worth living? It all depends on the liver.
~ William James

The liver processes practically everything that comes into the body. It is estimated that the liver performs more than 500 different functions in the body. One of its roles is to filter blood coming from the intestines via the portal vein. The liver plays a crucial role in detoxifying harmful substances by transforming them into non-toxic compounds. These compounds are then either excreted into the bile which is stored in the gallbladder until it is secreted back into the intestines, or the compounds are filtered into the bloodstream to be processed by the kidneys and eliminated via urination.

The liver is also involved in regulating glucose levels and hormones, and in producing cholesterol. If the liver is overwhelmed with the amount of chemical toxins that are pouring in, it will make a packet of fatty cholesterol and insert the offending chemical into the center of the fat. This way the toxin is well-insulated and cannot damage the body. Sometimes, the liver cannot eliminate all this toxic fat, and the person ends up with a fatty liver. The American Liver Foundation estimates that over half of the population age 50 and older have fatty livers. Research has proven a direct correlation between fatty liver and Type II diabetes.

Liver issues can cause constipation, flushing of the face, hot flashes, headaches, and feeling groggy and sluggish. And yes, men can get hot flashes too! An overtaxed liver will cause food allergies and other sensitivities, such as chemical sensitivities and hay-fever. High cholesterol levels, hormonal imbalances, hypoglycemia, insomnia, intestinal gas, and bloating can also be related to a congested liver.

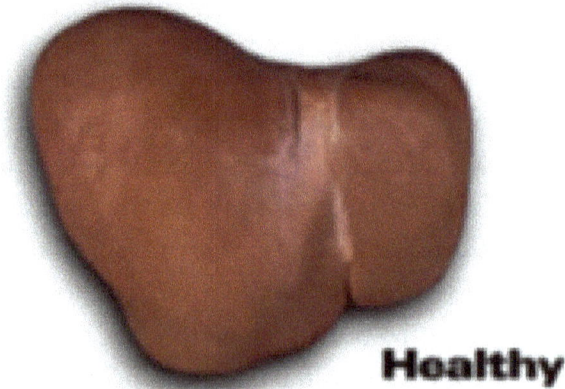

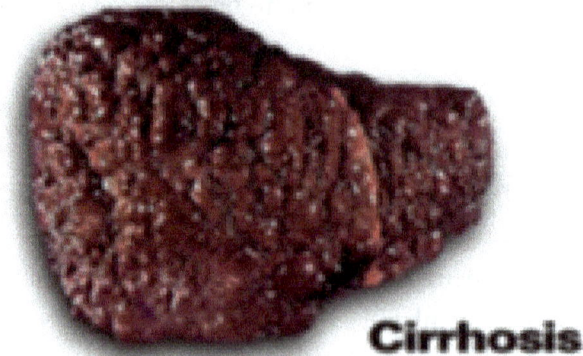

Healthy

Cirrhosis

Here we see the difference between a healthy liver and one with cirrhosis. We definitely want ours to look like the one on the top.

The gallbladder receives bile from the liver. Bile is stored in the gallbladder until it is needed for digestion. When we eat, the gallbladder contracts, causing bile to travel down the bile duct and into the intestinal tract. If you can live without your gallbladder, then why is it even important? Without the gallbladder, the liver cannot secrete enough bile to digest a full meal. Bile enters into the small intestines, breaking down large fat globules into smaller fatty acids, which are able to be absorbed. It also neutralizes stomach acid, which has been secreted into the small intestines along with food, so it does not damage the tender lining of the intestines. Bile stimulates the intestines to move, and gives feces its dark brown color. If the feces is light brown, bile is not making its way into the intestinal tract. Bile must be properly stored and released in the right amount and at the right time in order to prevent intestinal issues, such as heartburn, constipation, or diarrhea, from developing.

Gallstones are one of the biggest threats to a healthy gallbladder.

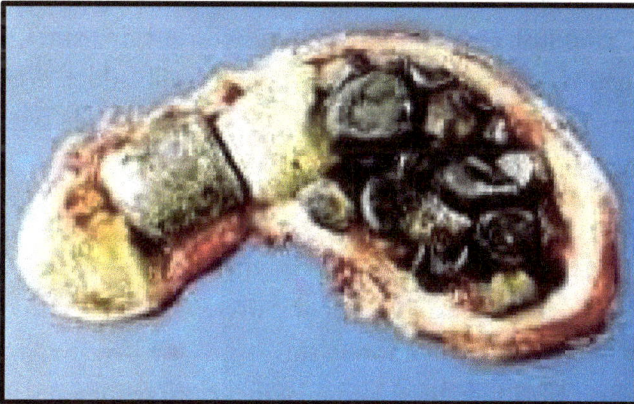

This is a picture of a gallbladder filled with stones.

The bile duct, not shown in this picture, would be a tube located to the far left end of the narrower part. Bile should be able to flow out of the gallbladder through the bile duct. You can see two huge marshmallow-shaped stones blocking the entry of where the bile duct would be, effectively stopping the flow of bile.

Bile from the liver can become thick like sludge, usually because of ingesting too much of the wrong types of fats. The gallbladder is supposed to contract, much like your bladder, to expel bile at the right time. When the gallbladder has been strained from pushing against thickened bile, it can become weak. A weak gallbladder will be unable to excrete the bile, which collects into gallstones, causing the gallbladder to become enlarged.

There are two main types of gallstones: cholesterol and pigment stones. Cholesterol stones are usually yellow-green and are made primarily of hardened cholesterol or bad fats. They account for about 80% of gallstones. Pigment stones are small, dark stones made of bilirubin. Gallstones can be as small as a grain of sand or as large as a golf ball. The gallbladder can also develop just one large stone, hundreds of tiny stones, or a combination of the two. Removing the gallbladder doesn't actually solve the problem. Instead, the thickened bile stays in the liver, where it creates stones that are stored in the liver instead of the gallbladder.

Another possible liver ailment is when parasites, called liver flukes, travel into the gallbladder and liver, where they can plug up the bile duct. I will address this issue later. Yeast can also infect the gallbladder, liver, and bile duct causing inflammation and pain.

Some common symptoms of gallbladder issues are: pain or spasms under the right rib cage—especially after eating fatty foods, severe upper abdominal pain, pain radiating around to the back or to the right shoulder; nausea, vomiting, gas, burping or belching, and heartburn. Although the medical solution for a congested or low functioning gallbladder is to take it out, you may want to consider doing a gallbladder cleanse instead.

Digestive enzymes are helpful to the liver and gallbladder. Most people around the age of 45 to 50 start running low on digestive enzymes, mostly because of an overly processed diet. Enzymes are abundant in raw or lightly steamed vegetables and fruits. Enzymes are critical for breaking down food and for carrying nutrients to wherever they are needed. Enzymes can be extremely helpful for people experiencing food allergies. Here is a quick run-down of the main digestive enzymes and what they do: hydrochloric acid and protease work together in the stomach to break apart proteins, amylase breaks down carbohydrates; lipase breaks down fats and oils. Lactase breaks down lactose from dairy; *alpha galactosidase* (guh-lak-tow-suh-days) helps break down the gassy part of beans and cruciferous vegetables; and cellulase breaks down fiber.

***

Some of my favorite products to use for a stone flush include:

- Lecithin (phosphatidylcholine) and hydrangea (*Hydrangea Macrophylla*) when combined, make an excellent liver and gallbladder stone cleanse that is safe, gentle and effective.

Lecithin is actually what the liver itself makes to break up stones.

- Milk Thistle (*Silybum Marianum*) is another great herb to use. Thirty years of laboratory and clinical research has shown that milk thistle is a balancer, which means it can stimulate a lazy liver, or calm down a hot or overly stimulated liver. Milk thistle protects the liver against chemical poisoning, protects cell membranes, and prevents toxic damage to liver cells. It increases glutathione which helps the liver detoxify chemicals. It facilitates cellular regeneration of damaged liver tissue, and also has anti-carcinogenic properties for the liver. It is very helpful in hepatitis, jaundice, liver inflammation, and cirrhosis of the liver.

- Dandelion (*Taraxacum*) is a common lawn "pest" that could feed a nation! Dandelion has been used in Chinese and European cultures for centuries for combating liver disease. It has a multitude of nutrients that help the liver filter out toxins and purify the blood. Dandelion increases bile secretion in the liver and inhibits bile duct inflammation, cirrhosis, gallstones, hepatitis, and jaundice. It has been used to treat acne, eczema, and gout. Dandelion has a high mineral content and actually contains more beta-carotene (Vitamin A) than carrots.

- Yellow dock (*Rumex Crispus*) helps cleanse the liver and blood. It has long been used by Native Americans as a liver tonic, especially for jaundice. Compared to other herbs, yellow dock has one of the most prominent reputations for clearing skin problems.

- Chickweed (*Stellaria Media*) is another favorite and can be very helpful for a fatty liver.

There are some great essential oils that have been shown to help liver and gallbladder issues. Typically, anything that will support the gallbladder, also supports the liver. In addition, it helps to use a castor oil pack by pouring castor oil onto a piece of cotton, flannel or wool and soaking it completely. Then add a few drops of essential oils. Place the cloth over your liver. Place a hot water bottle or heating pad over this and keep it in place for 45 to 60 minutes, or less if you find your skin is sensitive. You can cover the cloth with a piece of plastic such as saran wrap if you want to keep the oil off of the hot water bottle or heating pad.

- Grapefruit (*Citrus Paradisi*) can be used internally or topically over the gallbladder area to help dissolve gallstones.

- Peppermint (*Mentha x Piperita*) has been shown, whether used internally or topically, to reduce spasms and dilate the bile duct. This can help stones be passed more easily.

- Fennel (*Foeniculum Vulgare*), when taken internally or used topically, has also been shown to ease spasms.

- Geranium (*Pelargonium Graveolens*) essential oil can be used topically over the liver. It has been found to help with liver detoxification, a fatty liver, and rebuilding healthy liver tissue. It has also been used to help clear jaundice and dilate the biliary duct, allowing more bile to flow from the liver.

- Helichrysum (*Helichrysum Italicum* or (Roth) G. Don) is a wonderful oil for the liver. It has been shown to help stimulate production and regeneration of new blood cells. It is also effective in detoxifying drugs and tobacco residue from the body.

- Myrrh (*Commiphora Myrrha*) has been shown to have liver-protective benefits. It has been shown to reduce scar tissue and inflammation.

- Rosemary (*Rosmarinus Officinalis*) enhances bile flow and can lower high liver enzymes.

- Ginger (*Zingiber Officinale*) helps reverse fatty liver and stimulates bile flow.

- Cypress (*Cupressus Sempervirens*) helps flush out toxins from the liver.

***

Nutrition that helps to maintain healthy liver and gallbladder function includes foods such as: fish high in Omega 3s (anchovies, sardines and mackerel), nuts, olive oil, brown rice, millet, barley, fruits, and vegetables. Cooking spices such as Garlic, turmeric, and curcumin helps to stimulate liver detoxification, while turmeric and curcumin help flush out liver toxins and repair the liver. Avoid foods high in fat and sugar such as: fatty meats, poultry skin, butter, cheese, lard, whole milk products, fried foods, and pizza.

***

The mind-body connection of the liver and gallbladder are very similar. Energetically, the liver is affected when we hold onto irritability and anger. We tend to be fault-finding with ourselves and others. We tend to become depressed and discouraged, afraid and defensive. We are usually feeling disgusted with something in our lives. We might not even really know what our life is all about and we just want to run away.

Affirmations for liver issues:

- *I have courage and I am strong.*

- *I deal lovingly with situations in my life.*

- *I am open to loving discussions.*

- *God is supporting me.*

- *I look for the good in things.*

- *I love my strengths and bless my weaknesses.*

***

When we have gallbladder issues, we are soured with life's toxins. Somewhere in our lives, we are embittered about something. Even though we feel things need to change, we lack the courage to take action. We become set in our ways — very self-centered and willful, yet with an undertone of self-rejection. As we reject ourselves, we also hold back love and affection for others.

Affirmations for the gallbladder:

- *I have the strength to meet life's challenges.*

- *I can move forward one step at a time.*

- *I am open to honest discussions.*

- *I embrace the lessons and strengths this life has brought me.*
- *I release past grievances and choose to love openly and courageously.*

11

THE URINARY SYSTEM

*The secret of health for both mind and body is not to
mourn for the past, not to worry about the future, or
not to anticipate troubles, but to live in the present
moment wisely and earnestly.*
~ Dr. Edward Group III

The kidneys are amazing filtering machines, cleansing about
200 quarts of blood a day. As they filter, they remove waste
from our blood stream and combine it with water to form
urine. From the kidneys, urine travels down through two thin
tubes called ureters on either side of the abdomen to the
bladder and discharges it through the urethra. Kidneys also
produce several critical hormones: erythropoietin (eh-ri-thruh-
poi-e-tin) stimulates bone marrow to make red blood cells,
renin helps regulate blood pressure, while calcitriol maintains
calcium for bones and normal chemical balance.

A major problem occurs when the kidneys develop stones,
which are hard objects made up of millions of tiny crystals.
Kidney stones poke, scrape, and tear the delicate soft tissue
inside the kidneys and in the ureters, bladder, and urethra. Not
only does this cause extreme pain, but it also sets the kidneys
up for infections, which can be caused by yeast or bacteria.
Multiple infections over time can lead to chronic kidney
disease and kidney failure.

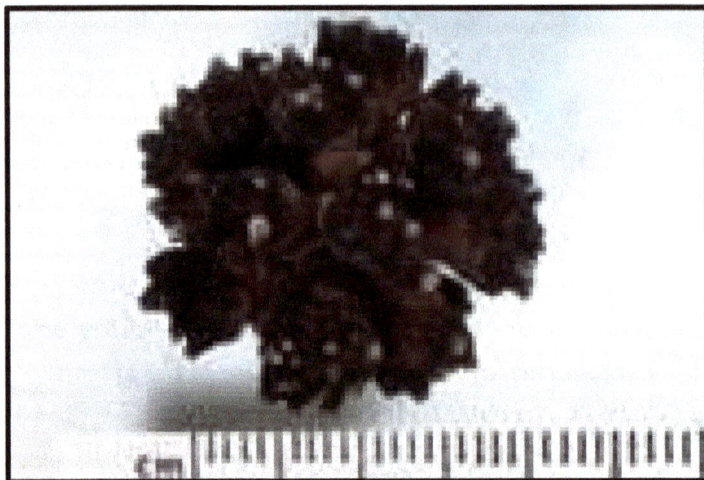

This is a picture of one type of kidney stone.

A diet high in foods and drinks that are acidic increases the risk of kidney stones. Acidic drinks include black coffee, black tea, soft drinks and alcohol. A diet high in animal protein will also cause the body to become acidic. The body, in its attempt to balance the acidity of the blood stream, will pull alkaline minerals like calcium out of the bones and use it to neutralize the pH. This process of leaching minerals out of the bones causes osteoporosis and bone spurs.

Once the blood is alkalized, the body then dumps this waste into the kidneys to be eliminated. If there is a lot of waste build up, kidney stones can result. Research shows that drinking just one or more soda drinks per day increases a person's risk of developing stones by 23% compared to those drinking less than one soda per week. Excessive salt intake has also been shown to increase the amount of calcium in the urine, thus causing kidney stones.

Eating a lot of meat protein causes acidity in the bloodstream. A 2002 trial of those following a high-protein, low-carbohydrate diet — as popularized in such weight-loss regimens as the Atkins diet — found dramatically increased levels of uric acid and calcium in the urine after just several weeks. To clarify, some meats and drinks are a lot more acidic than others. A neutral pH is in the range of 6 to 7 on a scale of 1 to10. Eggs, fish, liver, and oysters are in the neutral range. Chicken, turkey, and beer are slightly acidic with a pH of 5. Beef, cheese, and black coffee are even more acidic, with a pH of 4. Lamb, pork, shellfish, black tea, and cola have a pH of 3. Almost all fruits and vegetables are alkaline. A good idea is to keep your diet at around 65% alkaline and 35% acidic foods.

***

Some herbs that work well for the kidneys include:

- Hydrangea (*Hydrangea Macrophylla*) is amazing for helping dissolve kidney stones, along with other calcifications throughout the body.

- Uva Ursi (*Arctostaphylos Uva-Ursi*), also known as bearberry, soothes and tightens inflamed tissues, neutralizes urine acidity, promotes urine flow, and acts as an antiseptic and muscle relaxant specific to the urinary tract. Uva Ursi is especially helpful for cases of cystitis, acute and chronic inflammation of the bladder, and urethra. Uva Ursi is also a trichomonacide, which means it kills the bladder worm called trichomonas vaginalis. It can also prevent and dissolve both kidney stones and gallstones.

- Marsh Mallow (*Althaea Officinalis*) has been used in healing for around 2,500 years. It is helpful for almost any condition affecting the urinary system, including: cystitis, frequent urination, incontinence, painful urination, and urinary tract infections.

- Cornsilk (*Stigma Maydis*) is one of the best natural remedies for bladder, kidney, and prostate problems. Cornsilk relaxes and soothes irritated mucous membranes lining the bladder and urinary tubules. Cornsilk is extremely soothing for burning or painful urination. It also helps with difficulty in starting urination, which is common in prostate disorders. It helps with gouty arthritis, and has been used to stop bedwetting in children.

***

Essential oils can also be very beneficial for the kidneys. Once an essential oil enters the bloodstream, it can have a profound effect on the kidneys, since our blood passes through them twice every hour. However, some essential oils can produce kidney toxicity. These include wintergreen, birch, camphor, eucalyptus, tea tree, pennyroyal, thyme and oregano. Signs of kidney toxicity from essential oils include decreased urine output, swelling (fluid retention), fatigue, nausea and vomiting, confusion, and abdominal pain. To be safe, do not ingest these oils unless under medical supervision; dilute them at a rate of one drop of essential oil to 5 drops of carrier oil, and do not use them continuously over an extended period of time.

Some oils that are helpful for the kidneys include:

- Lemon (*Citrus Limon*) and Geranium (*Pelargonium Graveolens*) help decrease kidney calcifications.

- Eucalyptus (*Eucalyptus Radiata*), used topically, helps with pain.

- Rosemary (*Rosmarinus Officinalis*) used internally or topically, or both, helps with infections.

- Juniper Berry (*Juniperus Communis*) increases circulation through the kidneys and helps with kidney stones.

- Fennel (*Foeniculum Vulgare*), Cypress (*Cupressus Sempervirens*), and Rosemary (*Rosemarinus Officinalis*) are diuretics that increase the amount of water eliminated through the kidneys, helping with water retention.

- Sandalwood (*Santalum Album*), Juniper berry (*Juniperus Communis*), Geranium (*Pelargonium Graveolens*), Cypress (*Cupressus Sempervirens*), Cedarwood (*Juniperus Virginiana*), and Chamomile (*Chamaemelum Nobile* or *Anthemis Nobilis*) are helpful for kidneys, urinary tract infections, and cystitis.

Please note: apple and cranberry juices contain oxalates, which have been associated with a higher risk for calcium stones. Therefore, cranberry juice can help prevent and heal urinary tract infections, but should not be used for an extended period of time. In one study, just one 8-ounce cup of cranberry juice per day increased the risk for forming stones by 44%.

Most importantly — drink plenty of water! Many sources say between 47% and 75% of people are chronically dehydrated. How much you should drink varies greatly by individual. How much you exercise and sweat, or whether you live in a dry or moist climate, can make a huge difference in the amount of water your body needs. The Mayo Clinic recommends drinking 15.5 cups (3.7 liters) daily for men or 11.5 cups (2.7 liters) daily for women. Definitely avoid sodas, caffeine, and salty foods. Most sodas are high in caffeine — a diuretic that causes chronic dehydration, and one of the most common causes of kidney stone formation. Foods that are high in sodium cause your body to secrete more calcium in the urine, also promoting kidney stones.

For those with kidney issues, it is wise to consume a diet composed of 75% raw or lightly steamed foods. Kidney friendly foods include: pomegranates, avocados, broccoli, fish, tofu, squash, asparagus, parsley, watercress, celery, cucumbers, papaya, bananas, and tomatoes. Foods such as legumes, seeds, and soybeans contain arginine, which is beneficial for the kidneys. Limit your intake of animal protein.

A high animal-protein diet causes the body to excrete excessive amounts of calcium, phosphorus, and uric acid in the kidneys, often resulting in kidney stones. Avoid foods that contain or lead to the production of oxalic acid, including: beets, beet greens, rhubarb, spinach, Swiss chard, and vegetables of the cabbage family. Avoid alcohol, caffeine, chocolate, cocoa, dried figs, nuts, pepper, poppy seeds, and black tea. Avoid raw sugar, which stimulates the pancreas to release insulin, causing extra calcium to be excreted in the urine.

***

The mind-body connection of the urinary system is based around the need to eliminate something that is causing pressure in one's life. However, there is a fear of change and a belief that trying new things won't work. They have little self-confidence and believe that even if they get anything new, it will be destroyed or lost. They are living in fear, trauma, and shock. I was in this exact situation when I developed the kidney stones I told you about in my prologue. Thankfully, with a lot of courage, I found a way out of the situation.

***

Some positive affirmations for the urinary system include:

- *I am open to finding better workable solutions.*

- *I release and change until I am renewed and confident.*

- *It is safe to let go of _____.*

- *It is safe to grow and change.*

- *What I create inside of me can never be destroyed.*

12

THE LYMPHATIC SYSTEM

Wellness encompasses a healthy body, a sound mind, and a tranquil spirit. Enjoy the journey as you strive for wellness.
~ Buddha

The lymphatic system serves as the immune system's cleanup station and includes the lymph vessels and nodes, tonsils, spleen, and thymus. It produces soldiers that defend the body, such as: phagocytes (fa-guh-cites) that eat bacteria and viruses, helper T-cells that coordinate and drive defenses, killer T-cells that attack infected cells of the body, B-cells that destroy antigens and neutralize toxins, and memory cells that remember what we have fought.

A large majority of the lymph nodes are around the neck, armpit, and groin area. Because the lymphatic system does not have a pump of its own, it relies on the squeezing of muscles to pump lymphatic fluid throughout the body. This is one reason why exercise is so critical to our health. The lymphatic system can develop sludge and calcifications due to inactivity.

When the lymphatic system has problems, there may be swelling of the lymph nodes. The hands and feet may also swell. There may be excessive mucus congestion in the sinuses and the skin can also become very sensitive to touch.

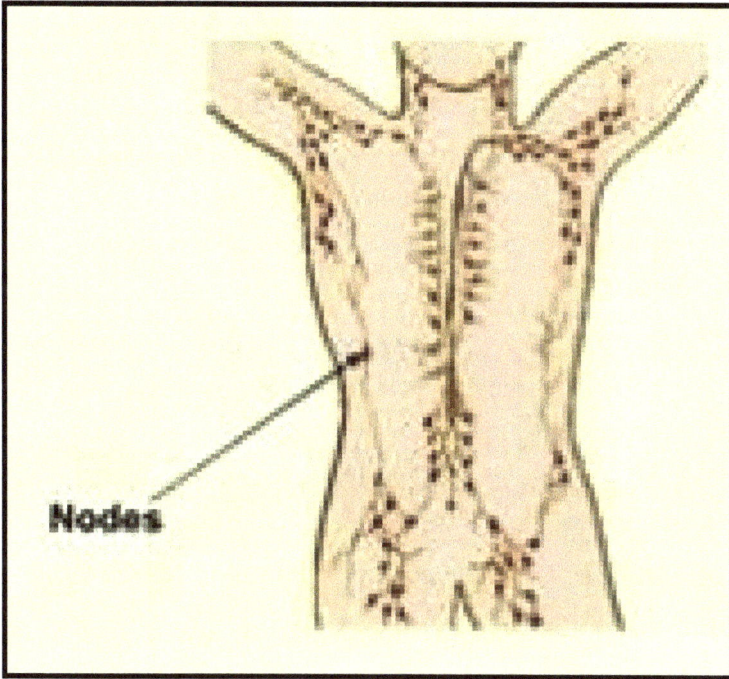

This is what the lymphatic system looks like.

Things that stress the lymphatic system are: illnesses that produce a lot of mucus from dead cells, an overgrowth of yeast or parasites in the body, and lack of exercise causing the lymphatic system to not get flushed out. One of the easiest things we can do for our lymphatic system is to gently bounce on a rebounder for 10 – 15 minutes a day. The bouncing does not have to be vigorous. Walking is also a great stimulator for the lymphatic system.

The lymphatic system uses a lot of minerals and needs adequate fluids to flush properly. Himalayan salt, sea salt, or electrolyte supplements are a good source of minerals.

Some excellent herbs for the lymphatic system include:

- Goldenseal (*Hydrastis Canadensis L.*) helps to strengthen the mucus membranes. It acts as a mild decongestant, relieving excess mucus while reducing the fever and inflammation associated with glandular swelling and sinusitis.

- Capsicum (*Capsicum Annuum*) helps increase circulation and enhances the removal of waste. It is useful against infections throughout the body.

- Red clover (*Trifolium Pratense*) has a long history of use as a blood and lymph cleanser. It has been used for chronic skin ailments, such as eczema and psoriasis.

- Yarrow (*Achillea Millefolium*) helps shrink inflamed tissues and enhances the removal of body toxins via perspiration.

- Cleavers (*Galium Aparine*) helps drain excessive fluid buildup and is well-known for its eliminative properties and action as a kidney and lymphatic strengthener.

***

Essential oils that are helpful for the lymphatic system include:

- Lavender (*Lavandula Angustifolia*), Rosemary (*Rosmarinus Officinalis*), Sweet thyme (*Thymus Vulgaris*) and Tea tree (*Melaleuca Alternifolia*), can help the lymphatic system produce white blood cells, which fight infection.

- German chamomile (*Matricaria Chamomilla*) and Roman chamomile (*Anthemis Nobilis*) aid in the detoxification process.

- Sweet orange (*Citrus Sinensis*) stimulates lymph fluid circulation.

***

Dietary suggestions to support the lymphatic system include: spinach, kale, chard, arugula, beet greens, broccoli, cauliflower, any kind of berries, salmon, sardines, sweet potatoes, beans, brown rice, turmeric, ginger, garlic, and rosemary. Make sure you are drinking plenty of water and exercising to move the lymphatic system.

If your lymph nodes are congested and swollen, or if you are having a lot of mucus, avoid foods that are mucus-producing, such as safflower and grapeseed oils. Avoid fried foods, processed foods, sugar, carbonated drinks, and dairy products. Avoid alcohol and caffeinated products, which are dehydrating to the body since the lymphatic system needs adequate water to drain properly.

***

The mind-body connection for people experiencing lymphatic issues is overwhelming sorrow. They have gotten to the point where they constantly wonder what's the use? They feel they are running on empty and putting out much more than they get. They feel they are literally carrying the weight of the world on their shoulders.

Positive affirmations that are helpful include:

- *When I need help, I ask for it.*

- *I pamper myself when I need it.*

- *Other people's baggage is not mine.*

- *I am centered in the love and joy of being alive.*

13
COMBATING PARASITES

Light attracts light. But sometimes your light attracts
moths and your warmth attracts parasites.
Protect your space and energy.
~ Warsan Shire

Now that we have cleansed the organ systems of the body, allowing it to effectively flush toxins, we are ready to go after some of the most disgusting things that most people do not even want to think about — parasites. Unfortunately, what you do not know can hurt you, and they'll suck the very life out of you.

Parasites feed off of other living beings. Human parasites include various protozoa and worms, which may infect humans, causing parasitic diseases. There are more than 300 species of parasitic worms that can infect humans. It is a misconception that parasites only come from polluted water or foods. It is true, some parasites come in this way, but we can also get parasites from fruits or vegetables that have not been properly washed, bathing in unclean water, walking barefoot in soggy soil, insect bites, inhaling the air from someone with parasites when they have passed gas, and from our beloved pets.

Parasitic infections are a crucial public health condition globally caused by intestinal helminths and protozoan parasites, particularly in developed countries, and are considered a primary cause of illness and disease. At least 30% of the worldwide population is infected with these parasites.

I worked with Dr. William Shroeder, D.O. for a couple of years while he was establishing his integrative health care clinic under the tutelage of Dr. Andrew Weil, M.D. A female patient came in presenting several complaints that led Dr. Schroeder to believe she had parasites. To his surprise, the results of her stool sample tests were marked as normal. Finding that hard to believe, he submitted another stool sample. He again received results that said normal. He was very frustrated and submitted a third sample to a different lab. When the results came back a third time as normal, he called the lab and said he was sure she had parasites. The lab then confirmed that she did have parasites, but there are about 30 parasites so common in stool samples that labs routinely report them as normal. As doctors, we were shocked and dismayed at such misguided practices.

Most blood-sucking insects are capable of transmitting infectious agents via their bite as they attempt to feed on human blood. In the United States, ticks transmit Lyme disease, Rocky Mountain spotted fever, Relapsing fever, Colorado tick fever, Babesiosis, Rabbit fever, and Alpha-gal syndrome. Fleas transmit plague and endemic typhus. Mosquitoes transmit malaria and dog heartworms. Triatoma (kissing) bugs transmit Chagas disease and head lice can transmit epidemic typhus. To make matters worse, female parasites of some varieties, can lay up to 300,000 eggs a day, once they are inside your intestines.

One of my clients was a nine-year-old boy, who was on five different medications from his psychiatrist. His health had taken a sudden, down-hill turn. He had been diagnosed with

ADD/ADHD, Obsessive Compulsive Disorder, and a few other psychotic behaviors. The boy was no longer allowed to attend public school due to the fits he would throw in class.

His grandmother brought him to me, and I was guiding him through this cleansing program step by step. When he was about 10 days into the parasite cleanse, something remarkable happened. His grandmother related that they were in a restaurant when the young boy came out of the bathroom yelling, "Gramma, Gramma, you have to come see this!" He grabbed her hand and pulled her into the men's bathroom. She said there, in the bottom of the toilet, was a florescent green worm wrapped around an egg sack! I asked the grandmother if she ever took her grandson to the beach, thinking that was the only place I knew of that fluorescent creatures exist. The grandmother said that they took him there every summer.

The next day, after giving him all of his psychiatric meds as usual, the boy fell asleep on the couch, slept most of the day, through the night, and was extremely difficult to wake up. They called his psychiatrist, got an appointment the next day, and explained what had happened. Over the next few weeks, the psychiatrist was able to wean the boy off of all but one of his medications. His attitude had completely turned around and he was able to get admitted back into school full-time.

There are many different types of parasites that can inhabit the human body, including: pinworms, giardia, hookworms, tapeworms, liver flukes, roundworms, heartworms from dogs, whipworms, and helminths — to name just a few.

Damage by parasites depends largely on which tissues are invaded by the migrating larvae, or the type of intestinal damage caused by adults. For example, after the ingestion and hatching of Ascaris eggs in the intestine of a new host, the larvae will migrate through the intestinal lining, through the lymphatic and blood vessels, through the liver, up through the right heart chamber, and into the lungs where they are coughed up, re-swallowed, and eventually establish as one-foot-long adults in the small intestine.

***

Here are some pictures of just a few parasite species that can infest the human body:

The first picture is of liver flukes. These parasites can infect the liver and gallbladder, blocking the bile duct and causing gallbladder failure.

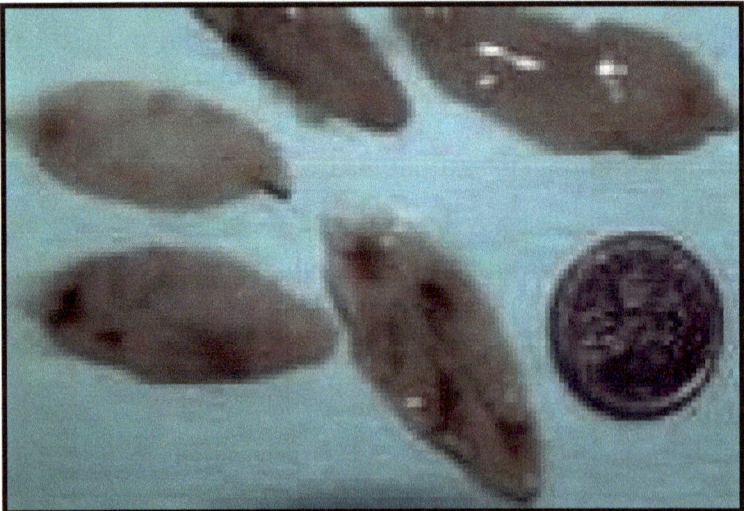

The picture below shows Ascaris. These live in the intestinal tract and can grow up to a foot long.

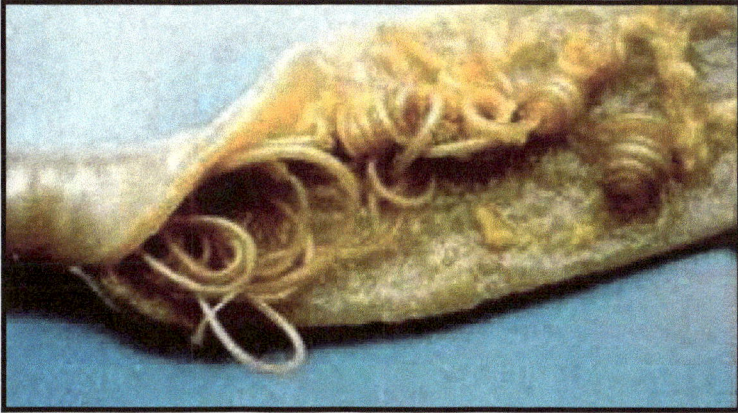

Below is a hookworm. Hookworms enter the soles of the feet when we walk barefoot in infested areas.

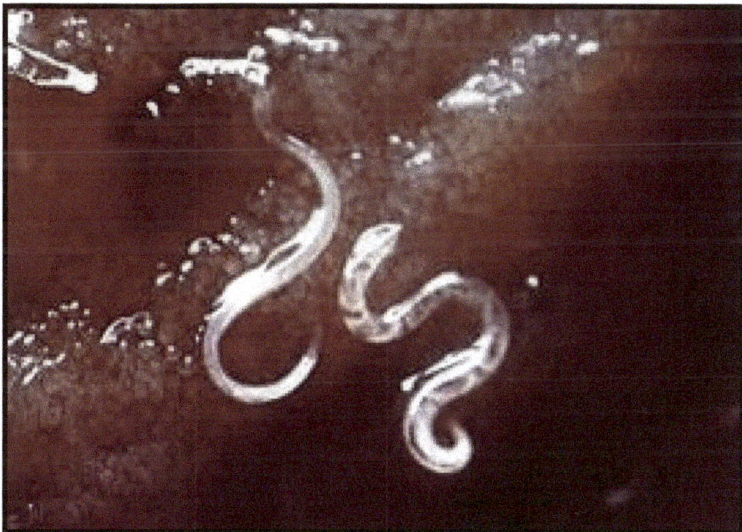

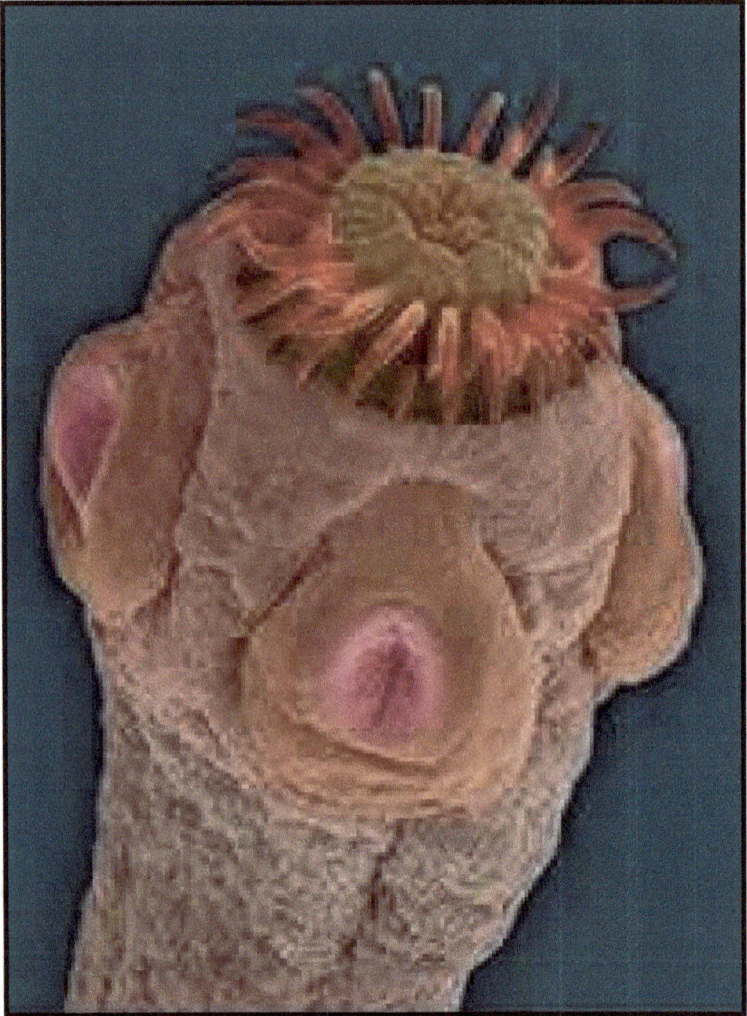

Tapeworms can grow up to several feet long. They release segments of their body which grow into new worms. Tapeworms can be very difficult to eliminate. If even one segment is left in the body, new worms can grow. Tapeworms can be extremely dangerous and life threatening.

I had an eighteen-month-old client who was not gaining weight. The mother and the pediatrician were very concerned, but the doctor could not figure out what was wrong. After surrogate muscle-testing, I told the mother I believed he might have parasites and recommended a parasite cleanse. About a week into the cleanse, the little boy was taking a warm bath. He had a bottle of milk with him, which had leaked into the warm water. His mother said he accidentally had a bowel movement in the bathtub and passed what she was sure was a foot-long tapeworm. He gained three pounds the following week and continued to gain weight until he was at his normal weight for his height. You may think this is a crazy story, but an interesting fact is that tapeworms are drawn to warm milk. One very old remedy for getting rid of tapeworms was to warm up some milk in a pan and sit on it. The tapeworm would be expelled as it migrated out of the body to get to the warm milk.

These are only two of the numerous stories clients have told me about the parasites they have passed. You can see how important it is to cleanse for parasites regularly!

Parasites live mostly in the intestinal tract, but can also live in the heart, lungs, liver, lymph glands, blood, and brain. The ones that live in the intestinal tract attach to the intestinal wall and eat the nutrients right out of your bloodstream. This means that they eat all the good stuff and leave the junk for you. Once they attach to the intestinal tract, they put out a chemical that numbs the intestines where they are attached, so the body no longer realizes they are there. This is why you may have a bout of diarrhea when you first get parasites, but it soon subsides — because the parasites have tricked the body into thinking they are no longer there.

Common health concerns related to parasitic infestation are: fatigue, malnourishment, food sensitivities, allergies, anemia, low blood sugar, weight loss or gain, an overall "blah" feeling, rectal itching, bloating or gas, reactive bowels, decreased attention span, or hyperactivity.

Parasites may also cause asthma, insomnia, eye pain, and rashes. Blockages may be caused by a large number of adults in the intestinal tract, liver, or gallbladder — leading to toxemia and death. Adult worms occasionally penetrate the intestinal wall or appendix, causing local hemorrhage and/or appendicitis. We really need to get rid of them!

***

I recommend performing a parasite cleanse two or three times a year, beginning just before the full moon, following a protocol of:

1. ten days on the products, then

2. ten days off, while using probiotics, and then

3. ten more days on the products,

4. another ten-day break, etc.

5. continue the pattern until the parasites are clear.

Starting a couple of days before a full moon is helpful because parasites are most active during this time. The ten-day break is needed because many parasite eggs will not hatch if they feel they are threatened. Also, if you are using oregano oil for a parasite cleanse, it can be very strong in the intestinal tract and can actually burn and harm the tender microvilli in the intestines, so it is best to not use oregano oil internally longer than 10 days at a time.

Do not be discouraged if you do not see any parasites eliminated in the stools. Many parasites, such as pin worms and rice worms, are extremely small and will completely disintegrate before being eliminated. Larger or longer parasites may look like strings of mucus when they are eliminated. Liver flukes may just look like dark or light brown patches of skin in the stool.

**

Some excellent herbs I have used for getting rid of parasites include:

- Black walnut hulls (*Juglans nigra*)

- Wormwood (*Artemisia Absinthium*)

- Raw pumpkin seeds

- Black walnut hulls and wormwood kill adult parasites and developmental stages of at least 100 different parasites.Cloves kill their eggs.

**

These oils have been found to have anti-parasitic activity:

- Oregano (*Origanum Vulgare)*

- Thyme (*Thymus Vulgaris*)

- Fennel (*Foeniculum Vulgare*)

- Lavender (*Lavandula Angustifolia*)

- Roman chamomile (*Chamaemelum Nobile* or *Anthemis Nobilis*)

- Clove (*Eugenia Caryophyllata*)

- Peppermint (*Mentha Piperita*)

You can use them separately or in combination. Hot oils such as oregano and clove should be rubbed into the arch of the foot to avoid skin sensitivity.

One of the most important and critical elements of a parasite cleanse is what we do after they are gone. Hydrochloric acid in the stomach is our first line of defense against parasites. It will kill them. Unfortunately, hydrochloric acid gets weaker as we age and some children do not have strong levels of it. Probiotics in our intestinal tract are our second line of defense. Good bacteria in our intestinal tract will eat parasite eggs and yeast spores in their infant state. But once they hatch, parasites will turn around and eat our good intestinal flora.

***

Lifestyle recommendations and dietary recommendations include:

- Wash all fruits and vegetables thoroughly to eliminate parasite eggs.

- Wash the tops of canned products before opening them. Parasite eggs can nest on the tops and crevices of tin cans so when you open the can, the eggs are spilled into the food inside.

- During the parasite cleanse, avoid raw or undercooked meat, especially: sushi, pork, lamb, and wild game. These undercooked meats contain a multitude of live parasites and parasite eggs.

- Avoid sugar! Parasites love sugar!

- Enjoy an abundance of: garlic, onions, chili peppers, pumpkin seeds, ginger, apple cider vinegar, yogurt, sauerkraut, and other probiotic-rich foods.

***

In the mind-body connection with parasites, people feel victimized. This may be in general about their entire life, or just in a specific situation. When parasitic energy manifests, it comes with a feeling of giving their power away. They may be in a situation where they are trying to get the "Good Housekeeping" seal of approval, but it never comes. Often, they have let others take over. They are not setting appropriate healthy boundaries and they are not expressing their truth or what they would really like to have happening.

Some helpful affirmations for people in this situation include:

- *I take full responsibility for my life.*

- *I take full responsibility for the decisions I have made.*

- *I speak my truth responsibly and lovingly.*

- *I am giving _____ the gift of truth.*

- *I set appropriate personal boundaries.*

14

ELIMINATING SUFFOCATING YEAST

Sometimes you just need to be selfish and take care of you.
If they love you, they'll understand.
~ Robert Tew

Yeast is the next cleanse on the list. A lot of people call it Candida, but Candida is only one type of yeast infection. The reason the yeast cleanse follows the parasite cleanse is because it is nearly impossible to control and eliminate yeast if you have parasites. Parasites are constantly eating the good intestinal bacteria, which is the first line of defense against yeast.

We breathe in yeast spores every day. They are literally everywhere, including the dust on our table tops. Yeast will thrive when our systems are overly-acidic from eating too many refined carbohydrates, such as: breads, sugar, rice, potatoes, alcohol, dairy, and cheese. Birth control pills and steroids, which raise hormone levels, also cause yeast to grow. On top of that, antibiotics kill our good intestinal bacteria, allowing yeast to get a strong foothold. The standard American diet, along with the volume of steroids and antibiotics being prescribed, has caused us to become more prone to yeast invasion.

Yeast can cause many common health concerns. It can spread throughout the entire body, by releasing spores into the bloodstream. Yeast can cause vaginal irritation, gas and bloating, mouth fungus, skin infections, rashes, joint pain,

Type II diabetes, brain fog, depression, fatigue, sinus pain, and cancer.

Yeast produces rhizoids with hook-shaped barbed roots that cut into membranes and cell walls causing pain and inflammation. If not treated, yeast will create a condition called Leaky Gut Syndrome, where the cell walls of the intestinal tract are so inflamed they separate a little. This leaves spaces between the cells where whole proteins can leak into the bloodstream. When this occurs, many food allergies develop because the immune system treats whole proteins like invading viruses and bacteria. The body then creates an immune response to the protein by putting out histamine, an inflammatory hormone. Histamine then goes through the entire body via the bloodstream and causes inflammation throughout the body, including the sinuses and the brain.

The following are pictures to give you an idea what yeast in the mouth, intestines and skin look like; below is the mouth:

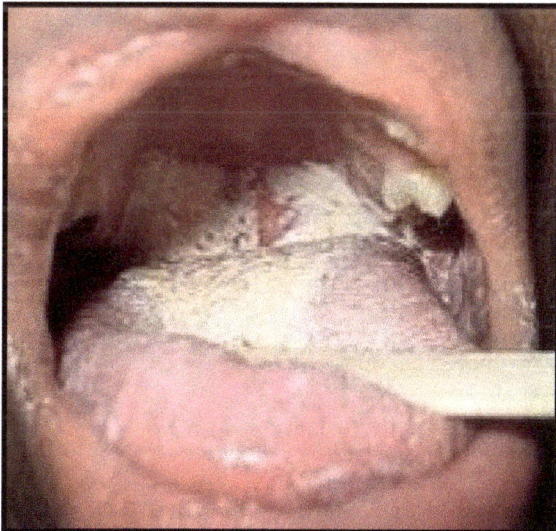

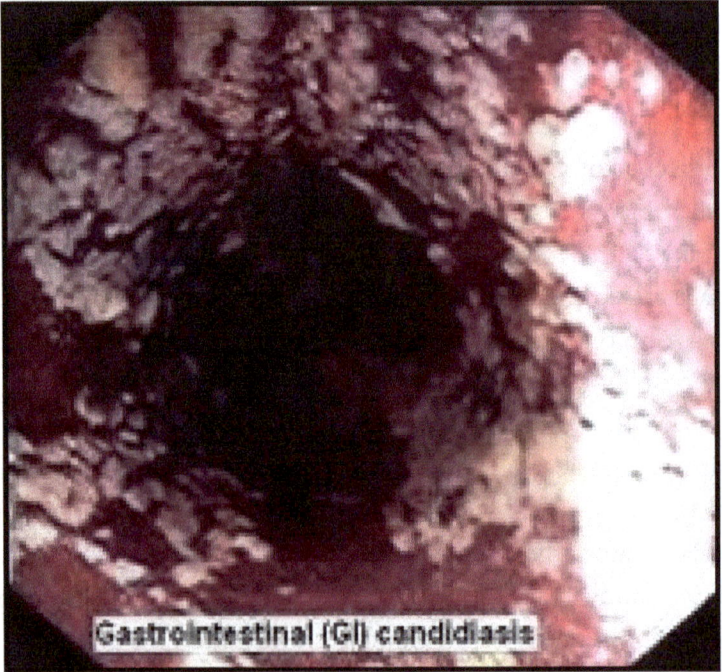

Yeast overgrowth in the intestines

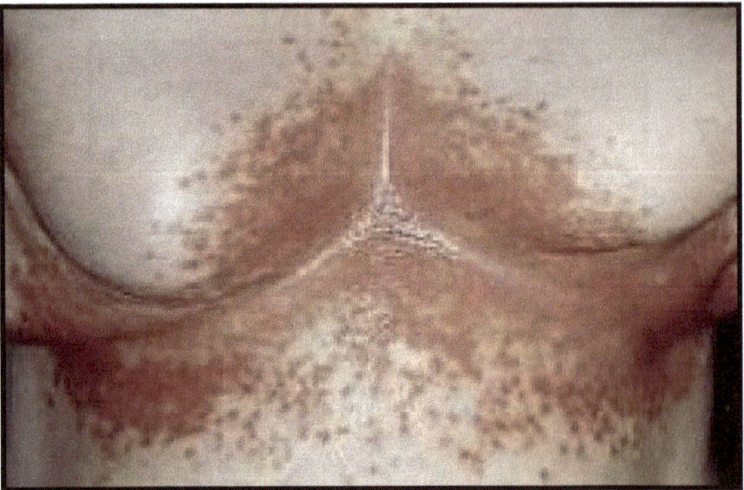

Yeast on the chest area

Some excellent herbal remedies for yeast include:

- Pau D'Arco (*Tabebuia Avellanedae*) is a broad-spectrum antimicrobial known for fighting bacteria, viruses, parasites, and yeast.

- Caprylic Acid (*Octanoic Acid*) is a naturally occurring fatty acid derived from coconut oil. The body itself makes caprylic acid to kill off yeast.

- Garlic (*Allium Sativum*) is both an antiparasitic and an antifungal.

- Selenium is a mineral that is listed as one of the most common nutrient deficiencies. It has been shown to inhibit the growth of yeast.

- Probiotics are critical for getting rid of and controlling yeast overgrowth. They are our main line of defense in our gut to keep yeast under control. Choose a high-quality probiotic that is protected from the stomach acid so they aren't destroyed before they can be helpful.

***

Essential oils that have anti-fungal capabilities include:

- Tea Tree/Melaleuca (*Melaleuca Alternifolia*) is a very powerful antibacterial, anti-fungal, antiviral, and anti-parasitic. It is useful against fungal infections, such as Candida, ringworm, and sinus and lung infections.

- Clove (*Syzygium Aromaticum*) is a powerful anti-fungal.

- Eucalyptus (*Eucalyptus Citriodora* or *Globulus*) is effective against fungal infections such as ringworm, Candida, and toenail fungus.

- Thyme (*Thymus Vulgaris*) is another powerful anti-fungal. It is also good for many other infectious diseases and has anti-aging properties as well.

- Oregano (*Origanum Compactum*) is a powerful anti-fungal and anti-parasitic.

If you are using oregano or clove topically it is best to dilute them with a carrier oil, such as coconut oil, so they don't burn the skin. To get the oils to circulate throughout the entire body, put a drop or two near a major blood vessel, such as on the wrists or the arch of the foot. While doing the cleanse, it is possible that the yeast will appear as a rash on the skin or in areas such as the ears, vaginal area, or bladder. If this happens, you can apply diluted oils topically to the affected area.

While you are doing this cleanse, dietary recommendations include avoiding: all sugars, refined carbohydrates, baked goods, starchy vegetables like corn and sweet potatoes, high-sugar fruits and fruit juices, alcohol, cheese, and milk-related products.

You can enjoy: broccoli, kale, Brussels sprouts, onions, tomatoes, citrus fruits, and blueberries. Chicken, eggs, fish, butter, coconut, and ghee are sources of good protein and fat. Fermented foods like sauerkraut, kimchi, and yogurt help build good intestinal bacteria. Gluten-free grains like oats, buckwheat, quinoa, and brown or wild rice, almonds, and flax seeds are also good. Steer clear of any other sugars and refined carbohydrates. Yeast feeds off of these.

***

The mind-body connection for yeast is feeling suffocated or smothered by someone or by a particular situation. People with yeast infections usually feel overwhelmed and very scattered. They deny their own needs and do not support themselves as they should. They may feel angry because they feel inadequate for the tasks they have or the life they have created for themselves. They have a hard time releasing past memories, harmful traits, and habits.

Like the parasite cleanse, those with yeast infections need to set appropriate boundaries. Good intestinal flora is like a healthy boundary in our bodies. We need to establish those same healthy boundaries in our personal lives.

***

Positive affirmations for yeast include:

- *I set appropriate boundaries for myself.*

- *It is ok to say, "No, I can't do that right now."*

- *I am able to responsibly handle the situations in my life.*

- *I lovingly accept my decisions, knowing I am free to change.*

- *I choose only to listen to loving thoughts in my head.*

15

BOMBARDING POLLUTION AND ENVIRONMENTAL TOXINS

By cleansing your body on a regular basis and eliminating as many toxins as possible from your environment, your body can begin to heal itself, prevent disease, and become stronger and more resilient than you ever dreamed possible!
~ Hippocrates

The last cleanse we are going to address is for heavy metals and chemical toxins. In a very scary study by the Environmental Working Group, researchers found an average of more than 200 industrial chemicals and pollutants in umbilical cord blood from 10 babies born in U.S. hospitals between August and September of 2004. The umbilical cord blood of these children harbored pesticides, consumer product ingredients, and wastes from burning coal, gasoline, and garbage. Of the 287 chemicals detected in the umbilical cord blood, 180 cause cancer, 217 are toxic to the brain and nervous system, and 208 cause birth defects or abnormal development. We used to think there was a natural fetal barrier that did not let stuff like this into our newborns, but now we know differently. Our kids are born already on the defense.

Where do these pollutants come from? They come from our outside air. They come directly from people in the form of perfumes, clothing, hair spray, etc. They come from chemical cleansers we use. They come from indoor pollutants such as: new paint, wallpaper, new carpeting, and furniture. When chemicals are released from new carpeting, paint, etc., it is called outgassing. Outgassing from new carpet is the worst during the first 72 hours of installation. However, new carpets will continue to outgas for approximately 5 years after they are installed. Pollutants also come from chemicals in our water supply. As if that wasn't enough, we also pollute our bodies with chemical hair color, nail polish and remover, and body lotions!

Amalgam fillings have been used for many decades and continue to outgas over the years, poisoning our bodies with toxic mercury. Although they are called silver fillings, the truth is amalgams have very little silver. One metal filling contains a combination of 50% mercury, 35% silver, 13% copper, and small amounts of tin and zinc. According to the World Health Organization, daily mercury absorption from amalgam fillings is 3 to 17 micrograms per day. The US Environmental Protection Agency states that a 150-lb. person can only safely consume about 6.8 micrograms of mercury per day, making the amount that is outgassed from silver fillings, in most cases, toxic.

More than 400 chemicals found in everyday plastic products have potential links to breast cancer, according to a recent review published in Environmental Sciences and Technology Letters by Silent Spring, a nonprofit research organization dedicated to breast cancer research.

A newer danger is found in the "forever chemicals" called per- and polyfluoroalkyl substances (PFAS). PFAS cannot be broken down by water, grease, oil, or heat. They have a strong carbon-fluorine bond, which makes them very difficult to degrade. They have been linked to cancer, high cholesterol, thyroid disease, liver damage, asthma, allergies, decreased fertility, and newborn deaths. Environmental toxins cause a lot of health concerns because these toxic chemicals mimic natural hormones and minerals in the body, confusing normal bodily processes.

There is also a great deal of electro-magnetic frequency (EMF) pollution from computers, cellphones, cell towers, electrical wiring, smart watches, earphones, etc. This type of pollution causes the electrons inside of our cells to become disrupted, causing oxidation and free radical damage. Our bodies are supposed to be grounded to the frequency of the earth, which is the Schumann Resonance of 7.83 Hz.

To help you understand Hz a little better and how they affect us, Hz is one cycle per second, MHz is a million cycles per second, GHz is a billion cycles per second. A computer screen emits 60 Hz of frequency. Cell phones emit a frequency of 600MHz to 53GHz.

Exposure to these frequencies can cause headaches, dizziness, tremors, loss of concentration, and memory loss. People with chemical, heavy metal, or environmental pollution overload may experience: chronic fatigue, rashes, muscle and joint pain, fibromyalgia, asthma and other breathing problems, dementia, Alzheimer's, autism, Candida overload, cardiovascular disease, thyroid problems, mood disturbances, anxiety, confusion, and irritability. People can spend years on unnecessary prescription drugs due to these health issues, which unfortunately just adds to the chemical overload in the body.

***

One of my clients was a 7-year-old boy who was diagnosed as autistic. The mother reported that the boy began having delayed developmental problems after receiving his MMR vaccination. He had never spoken a word in his life, only guttural sounds. With the help of his mother, I guided him through these cleanses. We soon saw some minor improvements in his behavior, but no improvements in speech. Then, approximately two weeks into the chemical detox, his mother came downstairs one morning to find the boy standing in the kitchen. He looked at her, pointed to the sink and said, "I want water!" The mother was elated! She called me on the phone, crying. She was astonished at what had just happened. Evidently, the boy had known the words all along, but because the neural pathways in his brain were full of chemicals and heavy metals, the proper connections could not be made. He continued to make steady progress at speaking more fluently, and within a year he was reading out loud and was rapidly progressing socially.

Many of our autistic children have become that way after being vaccinated. Their tiny bodies, especially their livers, can't handle the volume of germs, chemicals, and preservatives in the vaccines forced upon them at such a young age. The detoxification pathways of their livers shut down, causing more and more chemicals to continue to accumulate in their bodies. It is a sad and crazy thing we are doing to our babies.

Some simple suggestions to decrease your toxic overload include:

- Replace mercury-silver dental amalgams with ceramic ones.

- Drink clean filtered water — not bottled water.

- Eat organic, certified mercury-free seafood.

- Use an air filter in your home and spend time in rural, outdoor settings.

- Eat organic food — after cleaning it thoroughly!

- Choose to live a good distance from industrial areas.

- Use all-natural cleaning products.

- Use all-natural skin and hair care products.

- Get Electromagnetic Frequency (EMF) protection chips to wear and apply to your electronic devices.

- Slow the vaccination schedule WAY down, be mindful of which ones you choose to give, or eliminate some (or all) of them completely!

Natural, not synthetic, multivitamins and minerals provide some protection against many heavy metals. Heavy metals will occupy the same receptor sites as minerals. If the receptor sites are kept full with the appropriate nutrients, heavy metals entering the body will be more likely to be eliminated by the immune system, liver, or kidneys before they can lock in and damage the body. Chemicals are another story. Chemicals mimic hormones and can more easily slip past the immune system and occupy hormone receptor sites. Besides avoiding them, detoxing on a regular basis is the best way to deal with them.

Some herbal remedies include:

- Sodium alginate or kelp gum, which is derived from brown seaweed, has been shown to inhibit toxic heavy metal uptake in the bowels.

- N-Acetyl-L-cysteine (NAC) is a chelating agent in the treatment of acute heavy metal poisoning. NAC protects the liver and the kidneys against damage from heavy metal exposure.

- Magnesium blocks or nullifies the toxic effects of nickel. Magnesium is typically low in people with Multiple Chemical Sensitivities (MCS).

- Kelp contains algin, a non-digestible dietary fiber that binds heavy metals and radioactive particles in the intestines and draws these substances out of the body.

- Alpha lipoic acid (ALA) protects cells against heavy metal-induced toxicity. ALA has been shown to significantly decrease cadmium-induced liver damage. It is also effective in chelating mercury and lead from kidney tissue.

Essential oils that help to eliminate chemical and environmental toxins include:

- Lemon (*Citrus x Limon*) and grapefruit (*Citrus x Paradisi*) promote detoxification through the blood and the liver while stimulating the lymphatic system.

- Cilantro (*Coriandrum Sativum*) has been shown to be effective at eliminating heavy metals that can cross the blood brain barrier, especially mercury from amalgam fillings. It is also useful for detoxifying the pineal gland.

Recently, I treated a 72-year-old woman who was having a terrible time getting a good night's sleep. I instructed her to place one drop of cilantro on her wrist morning and night for about five weeks. Before using the cilantro, her pineal gland readings on the LIFE biofeedback machine were in the 20 to 30 range. A healthy reading is above 85. After using the cilantro for five weeks, her pineal gland was at 100! I asked her how she was sleeping and she replied, Like a rock! Needless to say, she was extremely grateful!

We need to consume organic food as much as possible. Even though it is more expensive, we either pay more for groceries now or pay more for doctor visits and intervention later. According to the Environmental Working Group (EWG) 2024 listing, the top 12 foods most contaminated by harmful pesticides are: strawberries, kale, spinach, collard and mustard greens, grapes, peaches, pears, nectarines, apples, bell peppers, hot peppers, cherries, blueberries, and green beans. A total of 209 pesticides were found on the top "dirty dozen."

The top 12 cleanest foods are: avocados, sweet corn, pineapple, onions, papaya, sweet peas, asparagus, honeydew melon, kiwi, cabbage, watermelon, mushrooms, mangoes, sweet potatoes, and carrots.

***

The mind-body connection of heavy metals/chemicals is one of damaging mental influences. These are man-made ideas that no longer serve us. It might be programming from our childhood by parents, teachers, siblings, friends, television, radio, movies, newspapers, or magazines. We find ourselves in a mentally polluted environment. We can feel really frustrated at how the "world" is controlling our thoughts.

***

Some positive affirmations for chemical/heavy metal toxicity include:

- *I am being guided by my own personal intuition.*
- *I love myself and honor my truth.*
- *I do not have to go along with anyone.*
- *My beliefs and opinions are important and valid.*
- *I do not have to buy into the crazy thoughts all around me.*

PART 3
THE PROCESS

16

THE CLEANSING PROCESS

The greatest wealth is health, because
without it nothing else matters.

~ Unknown

After detoxification and cleansing, many people experience a greater sense of vitality and well-being and are able to reduce or completely eliminate their prescription drugs. Learning to cleanse your body the proper way is easy, and you will feel much better once the job is done. However, you may still be wondering exactly how to proceed on these cleanses. So, I will give you one suggested protocol using products I have come to love due to their quality and potency. Remember everyone's body is different. I can give you a fairly accurate protocol of which herbal products to use. However, essential oils are a little trickier, as there can be so many that do the same thing. Generally, for essential oils, use two drops on your wrist or the arch of your foot, once in the morning and once in the evening for approximately four weeks. The best way to know exactly which products are right for you, how many per day you should take, and how long you should do the cleanse, is to muscle test yourself or have someone else muscle test you.

Over time, I have discovered that there is a specific order in which to do the cleanses to have the best results, in both the short and long terms. Just follow the instructions below.

STEP 1: COLON CLEANSE

Take Clean Start by Nature's Sunshine Products (NSP) as directed for 14 days and repeat if needed. Your goal is to have two or three bowel movements daily. Alternatively, you can use psyllium hulls and bentonite clay, or any similar product you have researched and are comfortable using. Put one teaspoon of psyllium hulls and one tablespoon of bentonite clay in a shaker bottle, add eight ounces of water or juice and shake vigorously until the clay dissolves. Then drink immediately because this mixture will thicken quickly and be unpleasant to swallow. Continue to drink as much water as possible during this cleanse or these products will not be able to do their job and you will become constipated.

STEP 2: CORONARY ARTERY CLEANSE

Take MegaChel (NSP). Follow the directions on the bottle, which will tell you to gradually increase the dose until you are taking four a day. Stay at four daily until you get a clear reading on your arteries, either from your doctor or by muscle testing. You can also use some of the oils that were mentioned in Chapter 9, or other oils you have researched and desire to use. Put a couple of drops of the oils on your wrist two or three times a day.

If you have mild plaquing, you may only need to stay on the products for a couple of months. If you have moderate plaquing, you may need to stay on the products for three or four months. If you have severe plaquing, you may need to stay on the products for five or six months, or even longer.

If you are muscle testing, a good way to make a statement is: If 100% equals an artery that is totally blocked, how blocked is the most blocked artery in my body? Is it at least 10%. blocked, 20% blocked?, etc., increasing the amount each time you ask. As long as the muscle being tested is holding strong, you know you are getting a yes answer. Once you get a weak response, which indicates a "no" answer, then you can ask about a lower amount. For example, if the arm stays strong at 30% but goes weak when you ask if there is 40% plaquing, then you can ask if there is 31% or 32%, etc. plaquing. Once you get a weak response in the muscle test, you know the answer is no and the previous value was correct.

Most people are able to do the colon cleanse and coronary artery cleanse at the same time. If you do not need to do either of these cleanses, simply skip them and go to the next cleanse. How do you know if you need them or not? Either get a test from your healthcare provider or do muscle testing. The more often you practice muscle testing on yourself, the more accurate your results will be. Testing yourself will ultimately give a much clearer picture of what you personally need for your body, while saving you a lot of time and money. Don't forget to follow the coronary cleanse dietary recommendations.

If you experience any discomfort or dizziness with this cleanse, large pieces of plaque may have broken away from the walls of the arteries. The products should continue breaking them down in the bloodstream and symptoms should pass quickly. If discomfort or dizziness persists, see your healthcare provider.

STEP 3: LIVER AND GALLBLADDER CLEANSE

If you have received lab results from your healthcare provider indicating you have gallstones, proceed with the cleanse. If not, muscle test to see if you might have gallstones. Gallstones can also be located in the liver, especially if your gallbladder has been removed.

The following products are all available through Nature's Sunshine Products:

- Lecithin - take six capsules of lecithin, either:
    - Two at breakfast, two at lunch and two at dinner, or
    - If you only eat two meals daily, take three capsules two times daily with each meal.
- Hydrangea - take six capsules daily in the same manner.
- Gallbladder Formula - take six capsules daily in the same manner

Continue this for about a month, or determine your appropriate length of time by muscle testing. You can also use a combination of essential oils listed in the liver/gallbladder section for an appropriate length of time. Follow the dietary recommendations described in Chapter 10. If you experience any discomfort during this cleanse, you can take some extra magnesium to help relax and open the biliary duct. You can also use a castor oil pack over the liver/gallbladder area, or take a warm, relaxing bath. If discomfort persists, see your healthcare provider.

STEP 4: KIDNEY CLEANSE

It is more accurate to call it a kidney stone cleanse. If you do not have a test from your healthcare practitioner confirming you have kidney stones, muscle test to see if you might need to do this cleanse. Keep in mind the limitations of medical tests. I have had a few clients whose doctors said the x-rays did not show any kidney stones, but they decided to do the cleanse anyway. During that time, they passed substances that their doctor verified were, indeed, kidney stones.

A suggested protocol for this cleanse is:

- Hydrangea - take six capsules. You can either take:

  - Two with breakfast, two with lunch and two with dinner, or

  - If you only eat two meals a day, take three with each meal.

- Cornsilk - take six capsules daily in the same manner.

You can also use some of the essential oils listed in Chapter 11. You can either apply two drops of each near a blood vessel on the wrist or the arch of the foot, or you can ingest them in a capsule or in water. Either method should be employed three times daily.

It is also a good idea to take Combination Potassium (NSP) during this time as well. This is a plant-based potassium supplement that helps flush the kidneys. Continue this process for at least a month, or until you get a clear reading from your healthcare provider, or by muscle testing. If you have discomfort during this cleanse, drink as much lemon water as possible to help any possible kidney stones continue to dissolve.

Some people may experience achiness in their mid-back, on either side of their spine in the kidney area. They may also experience sharp pains in the ureters on either side of the lower abdomen. Some women mistake this pain as ovulation pain, which can feel very similar. Most women easily eject the stones once they pass into the bladder. For men, it can be a little more difficult. Hopefully, with these herbal products, the stones will be completely softened before they are eliminated, so they can be passed without any discomfort.

If you are urinating through a fine mesh strainer and the stones have not been completely dissolved, you may see what looks like soft squishy globules. During the first part of the cleanse, you may notice your urine looks cloudy. This is typically due to sludge or unformed stones being released from the kidneys. As you progress through the cleanse, your urine will increase in clarity until it is completely clear. Follow the dietary recommendations in Chapter 11 and drink plenty of water. Most people can do the gallbladder/liver cleanse and kidney cleanse together, if they need both.

STEP 5: LYMPHATIC CLEANSE

Use the product from NSP called Lymphatic Drainage at ¼ teaspoon, twice daily. You may also choose some of the essential oils in Chapter 12. You can use two drops of each oil, two to three times daily. If you know specific lymph nodes are swollen, apply the oils directly to the skin above the affected nodes. When massaging lymph nodes, always massage from under the chin towards the spine, from the neck towards the chest, under the arms towards the chest, and from the legs or groin up towards the belly. The lymphatic cleanse is definitely a good cleanse to do when you are experiencing a mucous-producing illness, and can be done in conjunction with the liver/gallbladder and kidney cleanses. You should not have any discomfort at all during this cleanse. Your lymphatic system definitely needs to be clear before proceeding with the next three cleanses.

Using a binding agent is beneficial during these last three cleanses. A binder bonds with toxins to ensure the toxins are eliminated and are not re-absorbed in the intestinal tract. A few great binders are: activated charcoal, chlorella, pectin, and bentonite clay. Use them during the cleanses according to package instructions.

STEP 6: PARASITE CLEANSE

You should not combine this cleanse with any other one except the lymphatic cleanse.

Try to time the beginning of your first round of cleansing with the full moon, as parasites are more active during that time. Use the product ParaCleanse (NSP) as directed for 10 days, then rest for five to ten days, and then repeat as many times as needed until you test clear. You can also use GX-Assist from doTERRA, or a combination of some of the other oils mentioned in Chapter 13. It may also be helpful to combine some essential oils with the herbs, depending on the stubbornness of the parasites. Some parasites will be killed off quickly and some will take a lot longer. For example, it could take up to six rounds of a parasite cleanse to get a tapeworm to release and to kill off all of its body parts. Make sure to take a good probiotic during the resting period from the cleanse and for at least two weeks after the end of the last cycle. You can either choose a probiotic from doTERRA or Nature's Sunshine, which are both enteric coated, or one from a local store. Just make sure it indicates that it is enteric coated, protected from stomach acid or time released.

You may or may not see anything during this cleanse. Most smaller parasites, and even the longer ascaris, may come out just looking like strands of opaque mucus. I always tell my clients, if you don't want to know, don't look. Just get off the pot and flush it quickly! Only once have I had a client throw up parasites, and it was a very rare species. A Colonel in the Air Force, who had been stationed overseas, was having seizures and was extremely ill. Once he got them out of his system, the seizures went away and he was fine. He was very irate with his medical staff for not being able to figure out the problem and wrote me a very nice letter of commendation.

You should not experience diarrhea during this cleanse. If you do, back off of the amount of product you are using for a day or so. You may experience a bout of diarrhea if you are expelling a bolus of parasites, but it will be short lived. This may happen once or twice, but for the most part there should not be any other diarrhea or discomfort. You need to try to stay at the recommended dosage because if you don't, instead of killing the parasites, you will just irritate them enough that they will lay even more eggs than their normal 300,000 a day.

You may feel a little more tired during the first 10 days of the cleanse, but your energy should pick up afterwards. You may also experience a short head-cold or viral infection towards the end of the 10-day rounds. This happens because viruses live inside the bodies of parasites and, when they are killed off, the virus considers you their next host. So, watch out for any symptoms of infection so you can protect your immune system quickly with your favorite products. Mine are Echinacea/goldenseal liquid from NSP and On Guard from doTERRA, along with extra vitamins C, D, and Zinc.

Step 7: Yeast Cleanse

It appears that since COVID hit in January of 2020, yeast that thrives in the human body has mutated into something more difficult to kill. Because of this, you may need to use several products at once, or rotate a variety of products over a few weeks or months, depending on how well you stick to a clean diet and avoid sugars, refined carbohydrates of all kinds and dairy. You also need to use a good probiotic that is enteric-coated during the entire cleanse. PB Restore from doTERRA and NSP's Probiotic Eleven are both excellent choices.

A couple of really good products to use from NSP are Yeast/Fungal Detox and Caprylic Acid. Generally, the directions on the bottle are for a person that weighs about 150 lbs. If you weigh more, take a larger dose. You might also want to consider using some of the essential oils listed in Chapter 14 at the same time, or rotated with the other products. Apply two drops of these oils on your wrist or the arch of your foot, two to three times daily, so they get into the bloodstream and travel systemically throughout your body.

Yeast that breaks out on the skin as a rash, in the outer canal of the ears, or on the toenails is a little different. I had a very stubborn yeast infection in my right ear for months. I tried several different products, and even went to the doctor to have it cultured to find out what it was. The lab said they could not identify what type of fungus it was and the products the doctor gave me for a fungal infection did not work. The natural products I was using would work for a while, then the yeast would mutate and come back with a vengeance. What finally worked was a topical application behind the ear of doTERRA's Purify, followed by lemon eucalyptus, which helps cut the biofilm of yeast. I also dropped about seven drops of NSP's Colloidal Silver inside the ear canal and kept it in place for about 10 minutes twice daily. I was also using NSP's Caprylic Acid and maintained a very strict diet of protein, veggies, low glycemic fruits or sprouted grains, and absolutely no sugar or refined carbohydrates.

Yeast rashes have responded well to melaleuca and lavender used together. However, you may need to switch oils if the fungus mutates and is no longer responding to the initial treatment. If this happens, you can use doTERRA's Purify essential oil blend, or use Arborvitae and lemon eucalyptus. Lavender is always great to soothe the skin and stop the itching.

Fungal infections on the toes can be very stubborn. First, you need to file down the top of the toenail as much as possible without breaking the skin. Then, apply the essential oils so they can absorb into the area under the toenail. You can try tea tree oil, oregano, or clove. It may take three to six months of consistent treatment to resolve this issue.

You may notice additional mucus in your sinuses during this cleanse. Your lymphatic system may feel sluggish as well because the yeast is dying. If it does, you can start the lymphatic cleanse again and continue with it during the entire time of the yeast cleanse. Make sure you are moving since exercise stimulates the lymphatic system. You may combine the yeast cleanse with the environmental toxin cleanse. Together they can be complementary and more effective.

STEP 8: ENVIRONMENTAL TOXIN CLEANSE

A couple of really good products from NSP are Enviro-Detox and Heavy Metal Detox. Take them as recommended on the bottle. doTERRA has a complex called Zendocrine Detoxification Complex that is used together with their Zendocrine essential oil for this cleanse. It is also helpful to take a good binder, such as chlorella, activated charcoal, zeolite, silica, or bentonite clay. Using a binder helps keep the toxins from being reabsorbed in the intestines and reentering the bloodstream.

I would not recommend doing this cleanse if you are on a lot of medications from your doctor, especially heart medications. Do not do this cleanse during the first three months of your pregnancy. Also, be very cautious if you are on anti-psychotic medications, although this cleanse may be exactly what you need in order to remove the toxins from your system that are causing mental issues.

You may feel a little out of sorts emotionally when you do this cleanse because many environmental toxins mimic hormones. As toxins are pulled out of the cells and re-enter the bloodstream, they can cause some hormonal disruptions in your body. If you are a menstruating woman, do not be surprised if you have an extra period or a temporary disruption in your cycle. Men tend to feel angrier and women tend to be more emotional.

If you are feeling too emotional, you may need to slow down on the cleanse and only take half a dose, or stop the cleanse altogether for a few days and then resume. Be gentle with yourself!

***

There you have it! I have watched this process work again and again. Our air, food, and water are not getting any cleaner. Detoxification is a process we should all take more seriously just like changing the oil in our cars to extend the life of the automobile. Hopefully, cleansing on a regular basis will allow you to live a long, healthy, and vital life with many comfortable years to come.

REFERENCES

Balch PA, Balch JF. *Prescription for Nutritional Healing.* Avery; 1998.

Becker RO, Selden G. *The Body Electric: Electromagnetism and the Foundation of Life.* William Morrow & Co.; 1985.

Berger A. Quantum *Healing with the Biofeedback L.I.F.E. System.* CreateSpace Independent Publishing Platform; 2014.

Bock, Kenneth, MD and Stauth, Cameron, *Healing the New Childhood Epidemics -Autism, ADHD, Asthma, and Allergies - The Groundbreaking Program for the 4-A Disorders.* Ballantine Books; 2008.

Conroy VM, Murray B, Alexopulos QT, McCreary JB. *Kendall's Muscles: Testing and Function with Posture and Pain.* LWW; 2023.

Davidsson MF, Shaffer WL, Davidsson K. *Illuminating Physical Experience.* Holistic Wellness Foundation; 2000.

Diamond J. *Your Body Doesn't Lie.* Warner Books; 1979.

Dreher C. *The Cleanse Cookbook.* Christine's Cleanse Corner; 1997.

Frost R. *Applied Kinesiology: A Training Manual and Reference Book of Basic Principles and Practices.* North Atlantic Books; 2013.

Gattefosse R-M, Tisserand RB. *Gattefosse's Aromatherapy.* C W Daniel Company; 2004.

Hawkins DR. *Power vs. Force: The Hidden Determinants of Human Behavior*. Hay House; 2014.

Hay LL. *Heal Your Body*. Hay House; 2007.

Howard AB. *Herbal Extracts: Build Better Health with Liquid Herbs*. Blue Goose Press; 2005.

Kirschmann GJ, Kirschmann JD. *Nutrition Almanac*. McGraw-Hill; 2000.

Lepore D. *The Ultimate Healing System: The Illustrated Guide to Muscle Testing & Nutrition*. Woodland Pub; 1985.

Lincoln MJ. *Messages From the Body: Their Psychological Meaning*. Talking Hearts; 2019.

Marieb EN. *Human Anatomy and Physiology*. Benjamin/Cummings; 1995.

Moyers BD. *Healing and the Mind*. Doubleday; 1993.

Murray MT, Pizzorno JE. *Encyclopedia of Natural Medicine*. Prima Pub; 1998.

Myss CM. *Why People Don't Heal and How They Can*. Three Rivers Press; 1997.

Parker S, Fornari G. *The Body Atlas*. Dorling Kindersley; 1993.

Ross J. *The Diet Cure*. Viking; 1999.

Thom S, Thom A, Horst, Alexandra Ter, *Being Human: Exploring the Forces That Shape Us and Awaken an Inner Life*. Ad Humanitas Press; 2004.

Tisserand R. *The Art of Aromatherapy*. Healing Arts Press; 1997.

Tisserand R, Young R, Williamson EM. *Essential Oil Safety.* Churchill Livingstone/Elsevier; 2014.

Truman KK. *Feelings Buried Alive Never Die.* Olympus Distributing; 1991.

Versendaal-Hoezee D, Versendaal DA. *Contact Reflex Analysis and Designed Clinical Nutrition: A Healing Art.* Hoezee Marketing; 1997.

ONLINE REFERENCES

Fluoridation: https://origins.osu.edu/article/toxic-treatment-fluorides-transformation-industrial-waste-public-health-miracle (Note: article begins below photo.)

Microplastics: Tian Z, Ding B, et al, *Microplastics accumulated in breast cancer patients lead to mitophagy via ANXA2-mediated endocytosis and IL-17 signaling pathway.* Science Direct. https://www.sciencedirect.com/science/article/pii/S0269749124020384. Published November 17, 2024. Accessed May 21, 2025.

Parasitic Infections: https://www.dovepress.com/prevalence-and-predictors-of-intestinal-parasitic-infections-at-king-a-peer-reviewed-fulltext-article

Pineal gland: https://pmc.ncbi.nlm.nih.gov/articles/PMC6624939/

ABOUT THE AUTHOR

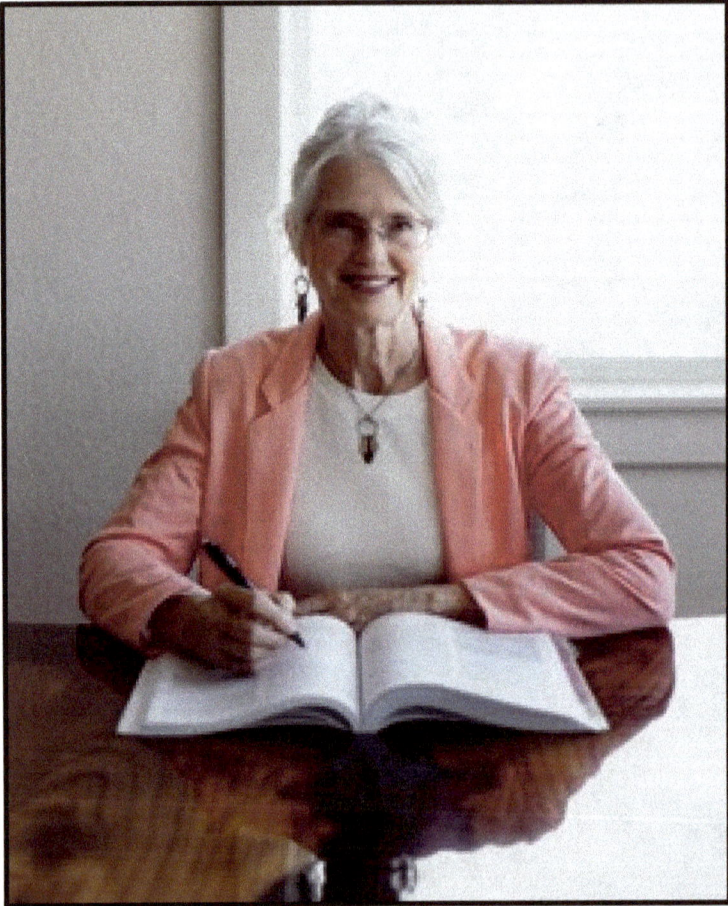

Cynthia L Maguire, ND, is a Board-Certified Traditional Naturopath with over 30 years of experience in natural medicine. She holds a Bachelor's degree in nutrition, a Master's degree in herbalism, and is a Certified Biofeedback Specialist (CBS) and Contact Reflex Analyst (CRA). Certified by the

American Naturopathic Certification Board, Cynthia has worked with clients of all ages—from newborns to the elderly —using gentle, time-honored methods to support the body's innate healing abilities.

Throughout her career, Cynthia has been a dedicated educator and public advocate for holistic health. She has taught for Memorial Hospital, Memorial Health Link, The Body Works, and Vitamin Cottage, and has spoken at numerous health fairs and community events. Her voice has reached wider audiences through magazine articles, KRDO's One Healthy Minute, and the Better Business Bureau's television series on alternative health care. She served on the Board of Naturopathic Physicians in Ohio, lobbied for health freedom in Colorado, and collaborated with Dr. William Schroeder, DO—an intern of Dr. Andrew Weil—to establish a pioneering integrative clinic in Woodland Park, CO.

With a rich career behind her, Cynthia is focusing her energy on sharing the wisdom she has gathered over decades. A passionate advocate of holistic healing, her mission is to empower others on their wellness journey through education and accessible tools.

You can learn more at healingessentialsguide.com.

www.ingramcontent.com/pod-product-compliance
Lightning Source LLC
Chambersburg PA
CBHW070923270326
41927CB00011B/2702